Clostridium Difficile Infection in Long-Term Care Facilities

Teena Chopra
Editor

Clostridium Difficile Infection in Long-Term Care Facilities

A Clinician's Guide

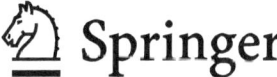 Springer

Editor
Teena Chopra
Wayne State University/Detroit Medical Center
Detroit, MI
USA

ISBN 978-3-030-29771-8   ISBN 978-3-030-29772-5   (eBook)
https://doi.org/10.1007/978-3-030-29772-5

This Springer imprint is published by the registered company Springer Nature Switzerland AG
The registered company address is: Gewerbestrasse 11, 6330 Cham, Switzerland

Contents

Contributors

Laurie Archbald-Pannone, MD, MPH, AGSF, FACP University of Virginia, School of Medicine, Department of Internal Medicine, Division of General, Geriatric, Palliative, & Hospital Medicine, Charlottesville, VA, USA

University of Virginia, School of Medicine, Department of Internal Medicine, Division of General, Geriatric, Palliative & Hospital Medicine and Division of Infectious Diseases and International Health, Charlottesville, VA, USA

Muhammad S. Ashraf, MBBS Division of Infectious Diseases, Department of Internal Medicine, University of Nebraska Medical Center, Omaha, NE, USA

Rishitha Bollam, MD University of Virginia, School of Medicine, Department of Internal Medicine, Charlottesville, VA, USA

Teena Chopra, MD, MPH Detroit Medical Center/Wayne State University, Detroit, MI, USA

Nisa Desai, MD University of Virginia, School of Medicine, Department of Internal Medicine, Charlottesville, VA, USA

Ellie J. C. Goldstein, MD Infectious Diseases Division, Providence St Johns' Health Center, RM Alden Research Laboratory, Santa Monica, CA, USA

Syed Wasif Hussain, MD Kings County Hospital, Brooklyn, NY, USA

Suny Downstate Medical Center, Brooklyn, NY, USA

Amar Krishna, MD Detroit Medical Center/Wayne State University, Detroit, MI, USA

Ravina Kullar, PharmD, MPH, FIDSA Expert Stewardship Inc., Newport Beach, CA, USA

Bhagyashri D. Navalkele, MD University of Mississippi Medical Center, Jackson, MS, USA

Justin Oring Detroit Medical Center/Wayne State University, Detroit, MI, USA

Introduction

Amar Krishna and Teena Chopra

Introduction

Clostridium (*Clostridioides*) *difficile* is a spore-forming, anaero-bic, gram-positive bacillus. It accounts for 10–20% of episodes of antibiotic-associated diarrhea and majority of cases of antibiotic-associated colitis [1]. The Centers for Disease Control and Prevention (CDC) categorizes *C. difficile* as an urgent threat responsible for about a half-million infections in the United States every year [2]. Infections caused by *C. difficile* can range from mild to moderate diarrhea, to fulminant and sometimes fatal pseu-domembranous colitis [3]. The national average mortality due to *C. difficile* infection (CDI) has also increased fivefold since 2000, likely due to the emergence of *C. difficile* B1/NAP1/O27 [North American pulsed-field type 1 (NAP1), restriction endonuclease analysis (REA) group BI, and PCR ribotype 027] strain with an estimated 15,000 deaths annually directly attributable to *C. diffi-cile* infection (CDI) [4]. In addition, about 20% of patients with an initial CDI episode go on to develop single or multiple recur-rent CDI episodes further complicating management [3].

A. Krishna · T. Chopra (✉)
Detroit Medical Center/Wayne State University, Detroit, MI, USA
e-mail: akrishn@med.wayne.edu; tchopra@med.wayne.edu

© Springer Nature Switzerland AG 2020   1
T. Chopra (ed.), *Clostridium Difficile Infection in Long-Term Care Facilities*, https://doi.org/10.1007/978-3-030-29772-5_1

CDI is 5–10 times more common in older adults compared to younger adults [5]; therefore, it is not surprising that older adults in long-term care facilities (LTCFs) account for significant burden of CDI. LTCFs may be defined as institutions that provide health care to people who are unable to manage independently in the community [6]. This care may be long-term residential/custodial care and short-term stay for rehabilitation or post-acute-care/skilled-care needs [6, 7]. The term nursing home (also called skilled nursing facilities) is defined as facility licensed with an organized professional staff and inpatient beds that provides continuous nursing and other services to patients who are not in the acute phase of an illness [6]. There is considerable overlap between the two terms (LTCF and nursing home) and the terms are frequently used interchangeably.

In the United States (US), there are approximately 15,600 nursing homes providing care to >3 million people each year, and on any given day, close to 1.4 million people reside in the nation's nursing homes [8, 9]. Close to 70% of the nursing homes are for-profit, and the overall occupancy is above 80% [8]. As noted earlier, residents of nursing homes (LTCFs) were mainly older adults. About 10% of the US population above 85 years of age reside in these facilities [8]. The population in LTCFs also have poorer health status compared to their peers living in the community with about 22% of residents having impairments in five or more activities of daily living (ADLs), 36% having severe cognitive impairment, and 34% severely incontinent of bowel and/or bladder [8]. In recent years, the acuity of illness of nursing home residents has also increased [10]. As CDI incidence correlates with the level of resident acuity and as the LTCF population is expected to grow due to aging of baby boomers, further increase in the number of residents infected with CDI can be anticipated in these facilities [11, 12].

It is estimated that about 100,000–110,000 cases of CDI occur in LTCF residents annually in the United States. This number comprises about one-third of healthcare-associated CDI [4]. About 70% of patients who acquire CDI in LTCFs are managed in LTCF itself without transfer to acute care hospital [13]. Studies also indicate that hospitalized patients with CDI are more likely to be discharged to LTCFs [14]. Both these scenarios place a significant burden on LTCFs. In addition, studies have shown that LTCF patients with CDI are at higher risk of more severe disease and mortality when compared to those who acquire CDI in the community [15]. This might be because B1/NAP1/O27 strain is the most common strain causing CDI in LTCF residents [13]. Infections caused by this strain of *C. difficile* is associated with more severe disease, more relapses, and increased mortality [16, 17].

Many factors are likely responsible for increased risk of CDI in older adults residing in LTCFs. Some of these factors include frequent hospitalizations, increased exposure to antibiotics, and presence of comorbidities [7]. It is estimated that 65–75% of LTCF residents with CDI had recent acute care hospital stay with majority of them being exposed to antibiotics [13]. Recent antibiotic use is the major risk factor for CDI. Apart from antibiotic exposure during acute care hospital stay, LTCF residents are also exposed to antibiotics while in LTCFs with majority of such use considered either inappropriate or unnecessary [18]. In addition, older age itself is a risk factor for CDI due to age-related immune senescence, poor/ineffective antibody response to infection, and less diverse microbiome [19–23]. Furthermore, LTCF residents receive care in a closed institutionalized setting, and healthcare workers in LTCFs provide care to multiple residents. Since *C. difficile* is mainly spread from hands of healthcare workers or the contaminated environment, there are greater opportunities for spread of *C. difficile* in the LTCF setting [3].

Due to the continued threat of *C. difficile* to LTCF residents, more needs to be done to address the problem. Surveys in LTCF setting has shown that recommended *C. difficile* related infection control and environmental cleaning practices are inconsistently followed [10]. Even more concerning is the finding that infection control is the most commonly cited health deficiency in nursing homes [8]. Despite the proven efficacy of antibiotic stewardship programs in reducing inappropriate antibiotic use and reducing CDI rates, there is lack of such programs in these facilities [10]. In addition, there are multiple challenges encountered by LTCFs in caring for CDI patients due to limited staffing, resources, and expertise which are not seen in acute care hospitals [24]. Such is the nature of the CDI problem in LTCFs that successful control will require involvement of multiple disciplines including facility leadership/administrators, physicians, pharmacists, laboratory, and nurses. Collaboration with regional acute care hospitals is also needed to obtain the resources and expertise for LTCF CDI surveillance, antibiotic stewardship, and infection control programs.

Various regulations, guidance, and support have come from national, state, and regional institutions in the United States to curb the CDI problem in LTCFs. The Centers for Medicare & Medicaid Services (CMS) mandated the establishment of antibiotic stewardship programs in LTCFs by November 2017 [25]. As of September 2012, LTCFs are also encouraged to report their CDI rates to the National Healthcare Safety Network (NHSN), and this reporting is currently mandated in the State of Nevada [26]. In order to increase NHSN reporting, establish CDI baseline in LTCFs, and improve outcomes, the Centers for Disease Control and Prevention (CDC) with CMS and QIN-QIO (Quality Innovation Network-Quality Improvement Organization) has established the CDI reporting and reduction project. This project has led to further collaborations with state health departments and regional academic institutions. In addition, CDC Infection Control Assessment and Response (ICAR) activity has developed tools to assist health departments in the assessment of infection control programs and practices in nursing homes and other LTCFs which can then be used to guide quality improvement activities [27]. Several other professional organizations such as Society for Healthcare Epidemiology of America (SHEA), Association for Professionals in Infection Control (APIC), and the Society for Post-Acute and Long-Term Care Medicine have provided guidance on the CDI problem and antibiotic stewardship in LTCFs [6, 28, 29].

Although several resources are available to address the CDI problem in LTCFs, there is lack of a comprehensive resource that addresses all aspects of CDI in the LTCF setting. This book aims to fill this gap and will provide comprehensive information on all aspects of CDI pertaining to the LTCF setting including epidemiology, risk factors, diagnosis, prevention and treatment. This book will also feature a chapter on LTCF CDI surveillance and role of asymptomatic carriers on CDI transmission and discuss the role of probiotics for CDI prevention and update on new recommendations regarding CDI diagnosis, treatment, and infection control. This book will serve as a valuable resource to physicians, LTCF leadership/administrators, LTCF nurses, infection control personnel working in LTCFs, and LTCF pharmacists. In addition, this book will serve as a useful guide to anyone who is keen to conduct research on CDI in the LTCF setting.

References

1. Bartlett JG. Clinical practice. Antibiotic-associated diarrhea. N Engl J Med. 2002;346(5):334–9.
2. Centers for Disease Control and Prevention. Antibiotic/Antimicrobial Resistance. Sept 2016. https://www.cdc.gov/drugresistance/biggest_threats.html. Accessed 19 Apr 2019.
3. Cohen SH, et al. Clinical practice guidelines for Clostridium difficile infection in adults: 2010 update by the society for healthcare epidemiology of America (SHEA) and the infectious diseases society of America (IDSA). Infect Control Hosp Epidemiol. 2010;31(5):431–55.
4. Lessa FC, et al. Burden of Clostridium difficile infection in the United States. N Engl J Med. 2015;372(24):2369–70.
5. Simor AE. Diagnosis, management, and prevention of Clostridium difficile infection in long-term care facilities: a review. J Am Geriatr Soc. 2010;58(8):1556–64.
6. Smith PW, et al. SHEA/APIC guideline: infection prevention and control in the long-term care facility, July 2008. Infect Control Hosp Epidemiol. 2008;29(9):785–814.
7. Chopra T, Goldstein EJ. Clostridium difficile infection in long-term care facilities: a call to action for antimicrobial stewardship. Clin Infect Dis. 2015;60(Suppl 2):S72–6.
8. Centers for Medicare and Medicaid Services. Nursing home data compendium 2015 edition. https://www.cms.gov/Medicare/Provider-Enrollment-and-Certification/CertificationandComplianc/Downloads/nursinghomedatacompendium_508-2015.pdf. Accessed 19 Apr 2019.
9. Centers for Medicare and Medicaid Services. CMS survey and certification group 2016/2017 nursing home action plan. https://www.cms.gov/Medicare/Provider-Enrollment-and-Certification/CertificationandComplianc/Downloads/2016-2017-Nursing-Home-Action-Plan.pdf. Accessed 19 Apr 2019.
10. AHCA. Quality report, 2013. https://www.ahcancal.org/qualityreport/Documents/AHCA_2013QR_ONLINE.pdf. Accessed 19 Apr 2019.
11. Laffan AM, et al. Burden of Clostridium difficile-associated diarrhea in a long-term care facility. J Am Geriatr Soc. 2006;54(7):1068–73.
12. Department of Health and Human Services, Office of the Assistant Secretary for Planning and Evaluation. The future supply of long-term care workers in relation to the aging baby boom generation: report to Congress. Washington, DC: HHS. http://aspe.hhs.gov/daltcp/reports/ltcwork.htm. Accessed 3 Nov 2019.

13. Hunter JC, et al. Burden of nursing home-onset Clostridium difficile infection in the United States: estimates of incidence and patient outcomes. Open Forum Infect Dis. 2016;3(1):ofv196.
14. Dubberke ER, et al. Attributable outcomes of endemic Clostridium difficile-associated disease in nonsurgical patients. Emerg Infect Dis. 2008;14(7):1031–8.
15. Karanika S, et al. The attributable burden of Clostridium difficile infection to long-term care facilities stay: a clinical study. J Am Geriatr Soc. 2017;65(8):1733–40.
16. See I, et al. NAP1 strain type predicts outcomes from Clostridium difficile infection. Clin Infect Dis. 2014;58(10):1394–400.
17. Figueroa I, et al. Relapse versus reinfection: recurrent Clostridium difficile infection following treatment with fidaxomicin or vancomycin. Clin Infect Dis. 2012;55(Suppl 2):S104–9.
18. Centers for Disease Control and Prevention. The core elements of antibiotic stewardship for nursing homes. https://www.cdc.gov/longtermcare/pdfs/core-elements-antibiotic-stewardship.pdf. Accessed 19 Apr 2019.
19. Loo VG, et al. Host and pathogen factors for Clostridium difficile infection and colonization. N Engl J Med. 2011;365(18):1693–703.
20. Kelly CP. Can we identify patients at high risk of recurrent Clostridium difficile infection? Clin Microbiol Infect. 2012;18(Suppl 6):21–7.
21. Viscidi R, et al. Serum antibody response to toxins A and B of Clostridium difficile. J Infect Dis. 1983;148(1):93–100.
22. Nakamura S, et al. Isolation of Clostridium difficile from the feces and the antibody in sera of young and elderly adults. Microbiol Immunol. 1981;25(4):345–51.
23. Biagi E, et al. Through ageing, and beyond: gut microbiota and inflammatory status in seniors and centenarians. PLoS One. 2010;5(5):e10667.
24. Jump RL, Donskey CJ. Clostridium difficile in the long-term care facility: prevention and management. Curr Geriatr Rep. 2015;4(1):60–9.
25. Centers for Medicare & Medicaid Services. CMS issues proposed rule that prohibits discrimination, reduces hospital-acquired conditions, and promotes antibiotic stewardship in hospitals. Available at: https://www.cms.gov/Newsroom/.
26. Palms DL, et al. The National Healthcare Safety Network Long-term Care Facility Component early reporting experience: January 2013–December 2015. Am J Infect Control. 2018;46(6):637–42.
27. Centers for Disease Control and Prevention. Infection control assessment tool for long-term care facilities. https://www.cdc.gov/infectioncontrol/pdf/icar/ltcf.pdf. Accessed 17 Apr 2019.
28. Simor AE, et al. Clostridium difficile in long-term-care facilities for the elderly. Infect Control Hosp Epidemiol. 2002;23(11):696–703.
29. Jump RLP, et al. Template for an antibiotic stewardship policy for post-acute and long-term care settings. J Am Med Dir Assoc. 2017;18(11):913–20.

Epidemiology of *Clostridioides difficile* Infection in Long-Term Care Facilities

Syed Wasif Hussain
and Muhammad Salman Ashraf

Introduction

Clostridioides difficile (formerly known as *Clostridium difficile*) is a Gram-positive, spore-forming, anaerobic bacillus. It was first described in 1935 as part of the intestinal flora of newborn infants [1]. However, it was not recognized as a major cause of pseudomembranous colitis until 1978 [2]. Over the period of decades, *C. difficile* has reached an epidemic state with increasing incidence and severity in both healthcare and community settings [3]. *Clostridium difficile* is the leading cause of healthcare-associated gastrointestinal infections and the most commonly reported pathogen causing healthcare-associated infections in the USA accounting for 12.1% of all healthcare-associated infections [4].

S. W. Hussain
Kings County Hospital, Brooklyn, NY, USA

Suny Downstate Medical Center, Brooklyn, NY, USA

M. S. Ashraf (✉)
Division of Infectious Diseases, Department of Internal Medicine,
University of Nebraska Medical Center, Omaha, NE, USA
e-mail: salman.ashraf@unmc.edu

© Springer Nature Switzerland AG 2020   7
T. Chopra (ed.), *Clostridium Difficile Infection in Long-Term Care Facilities*, https://doi.org/10.1007/978-3-030-29772-5_2

Because of the morbidity and mortality associated with CDI, CDC has called *C. difficile* as an urgent threat to public health [5]. Long-term care facilities (LTCF) should pay particular attention to this threat for several reasons. *C. difficile* colonization rates in LTCF have been shown to be higher than the surrounding community [6]. Similarly, transmission of *C. difficile* within LTCF has also been shown to be much higher than in the community [7]. In addition, the elderly residents of LTCF are at higher risk for getting *C. difficile* infections (CDI), and the mortality rates of CDI in this population are also higher than the mortality rates for community-associated and overall healthcare-associated CDI [8–11]. Therefore, it is important to review the epidemiology of CDI in long-term care setting.

C. difficile Strain Diversity in Long-Term Care Facilities

In the past two decades, the epidemiology of CDI has changed significantly worldwide [12]. Reports of increased incidence and complications of CDI from severe forms of CDI started to emerge from different parts of the world. This shift, at least in part, was linked to the emergence and epidemic spread of a novel strain of *C. difficile* especially in North America and Europe [12]. This epidemic strain has reduced susceptibility to the fluoroquinolone as compared to the previously found isolates of *C. difficile*. Later on, this strain was identified as North American pulsed-field type 1 (NAP1), restriction endonuclease analysis (REA) group BI, and PCR ribotype 027 (also known as BI/NAP1/027) [12].

One report showed that the overall CDI hospitalization incidence in the USA rose from 6.4 cases per 10,000 in 2000 to 13.1 cases per 10,000 in 2005 [13]. In addition to that, the age-adjusted case-fatality rate for CDI hospitalizations nearly doubled during that time period (1.2% in 2000 to 2.2% in 2004) [13]. Even though CDI incidence rate increased in all age groups, the rate of increase was much steeper in adults over the age of 65 with the steepest trend noticed in adults over 85 years of age [13]. The slope for the linear trend was 11.3 (95% confidence interval [CI] 7.6–14.9, $p = 0.001$) in adults over 85 years of age as compared to 4.8 (95%

CI 3.2–6.0, $p < 0.001$) among the 65–84 age group and 0.2 (95% CI 0.1–0.3, $p < 0.001$) among the adults aged 18–44 years [13].

In a study conducted during 2010–2011 in the USA, ribotype O27 strain was found to be the most prevalent strain among inpatients admitted from LTCF [14]. Almost three quarters (71%) of the CDI patients admitted from the LTCF were infected with *C. difficile* ribotype 027 strains and 75% with strains with high-level fluoroquinolone resistance. This was much higher proportions as compared with 34% and 44%, respectively, for patients admitted from home. Patients infected with ribotype 027 strains had a higher all-cause mortality rate and more intestinal inflammation, as measured by quantitative fecal lactoferrin [14].

It has also been noticed that when *C. difficile* is present in LTCF residents, multiple strains of the organism are often found in the facility [15]. In a single nursing home outbreak in the USA, where all clinical specimens were found to have ribotype 027, 21% of the positive environmental cultures had *C. difficile* isolates other than ribotype 027 [16]. The prevalence of these strains in LTCF may also vary based on the geographic region. For example, a German study looking into the prevalence of *C. difficile* colonization among nursing home residents found ribotypes 014 and 001 as the most prevalent genotypes that accounted for 30% and 20% of toxigenic isolates in nursing homes, respectively [6]. A study conducted in eight nursing homes in Hong Kong demonstrated that the residents were most frequently colonized by *C. difficile* ribotypes 002 (40.8%), 014 (16.9%), 029 (9.9%), and 053 (8.5%) [17]. Another study conducted in 2013 in a Belgian nursing home found ribotype 027 as the predominant strain even though ribotypes 078 and 014/020 were the predominant strains in the hospitals around that time [18]. The proportion of hospitals with the ribotype 027 strain decreased from 34% in 2009 to 15% in 2013 in Belgium. The authors of this study hypothesized that they may see a change in the nursing home strains in a few years as changes in the nursing home strains usually come later than the hospitals.

It has also been shown that as compared to the hospital and outpatient setting, the clinically indicated specimens submitted for *C. difficile* from nursing homes have higher prevalence of toxigenic strains (at least 2.5 times higher than either of the two settings) [19]. In the same study conducted in Southwest Virginia, it was found that the nursing homes have the lowest diversity of the ribotypes as compared to the inpatient and outpatient setting. Ribotype analysis of 190 toxigenic isolates was performed that included 56 inpatient, 69 outpatient, and 65 nursing home isolates. Only six different ribotypes were identified in nursing home patients as compared to 23 and 21 ribotypes for inpatients and outpatients, respectively. Ribotype 027 was the predominant strain and accounted for about half of the ribotypes identified in the nursing home patients [19].

Incidence and Prevalence of *C. difficile* Infection

CDI in the past used to be considered a problem for acute care hospitals, but more recent data clearly shows that prevalence of CDI is not only a threat for the hospitalized patients but also for residents of long-term care settings and everyone in the community [8, 20–25]. The estimates of incidence and prevalence of CDI in LTCF vary from study to study. Incidence rates may be as high as 3.72 cases/1000 resident days in the US LTCF, and prevalence has been reported to be as high as 3.8% of LTCF admissions [26]. These numbers might even be higher in the setting of an outbreak. Subacute and rehabilitation units of LTCF (where majority of patients get admitted from hospital setting) have also been reported to have higher incidence and prevalence of CDI as compared to the traditional nursing home units (where patients typically get admitted from the community or after failing inpatient rehabilitation) [27].

Based on active population- and laboratory-based surveillance across 10 geographic areas, it was estimated that 453,000 (95% confidence interval [CI], 397,100–508,500) initial cases of CDI occurred in the USA during 2011 [8]. The incidence was estimated to be higher among females as compared to males (rate ratio, 1.26; 95% CI, 1.25–1.27), whites as compared to non-whites (rate ratio, 1.72; 95% CI, 1.56–2.0), and persons 65 years of age or older as compared to those younger than 65 years of age (rate ratio, 8.65; 95% CI, 8.16–9.31) [8]. This particular study also investigated the origin of the CDI and classified community-associated infections as those CDI where the *C. difficile*–positive specimen was collected on an outpatient basis or within 3 days after hospital admission in those patients who had no documented overnight stay in a healthcare facility during the previous 12 weeks. The rest of the CDI were classified as healthcare-associated infections and further divided into three distinct groups: community onset associated with a healthcare facility, hospital onset, or nursing home onset. The national estimated incidence of community-associated and healthcare-associated CDI was 51.9 (95% confidence interval [CI], 43.2–60.5) and 95.3 (95% CI, 85.9–104.8) per 100,000 population, respectively. This accounted for an estimated 159,700 community-associated and 293,000 healthcare-associated CDI. Over a third (104,400, 95% CI, 94,100–115,800) of all healthcare-associated CDI cases were estimated to have a nursing home onset [8].

Another retrospective cohort study estimated prevalence of CDI in US LTCF by using the 2011 LTCF resident data from the Minimum Data Set 3.0 linked to Medicare claims. The nationwide CDI prevalence rate was 1.85 per 100 LTCF admissions (95% confidence interval [CI] 1.83–1.87) [11]. Older age, white race, presence of a feeding tube, unhealed pressure ulcers, end-stage renal disease, cirrhosis, bowel incontinence, prior tracheostomy, chemotherapy, and chronic obstructive pulmonary disease were independently related to "high risk" for CDI in this study.

The fact that some patients who developed CDI in LTCF may also have been exposed to hospital, ambulatory care, or community settings in the past few months before the diagnosis makes it harder to determine the setting of acquisition and presents a challenge in estimating true incidence of a nursing home–onset CDI. The reason for the uncertainty is that the studies have shown variable time interval for an individual to develop CDI after the exposure [28]. The range varies from less than a week to months (2–3 months). However, it has also been described that majority of the cases with a delayed-onset CDI have symptom onset within 4 weeks after the discharge from a hospital [28]. For the purposes of surveillance, the CDC defines the cases to be an LTCF onset if the positive *C. difficile* sample was obtained more than 3 days after admission to the LTCF [29]. However, the CDC further sub-classifies LTCF-onset CDI cases as acute-care transfer–LTCF onset if the stool specimen is collected ≤4 weeks following transfer from an acute-care facility [29]. Several studies have shown that majority (>50%) of LTCF onset CDI cases are diagnosed within a month after discharge from hospital [24, 30–33]. One VA study reported 85% of LTCF-onset CDI cases occurring within 1 month after transfer from the hospital [31]. However, a follow-up study in the same setting demonstrated that LTCF residents frequently acquired colonization with toxigenic *C. difficile* after transfer from the hospital [30]. Three quarters (75%) of initial CDI cases with onset within 1 month of transfer occurred in residents who acquired colonization in the LTCF. This result challenges the concept of classifying LTCF-onset CDI cases diagnosed within a month of hospital discharge as hospital associated. It is also important to note that antibiotic exposure in the hospital was identified as a potential risk factor for acquisition of colonization within LTCF in the same study which points toward the complexity of associating CDI cases with the hospital or the LTCF [30].

Colonization of Long-Term Care Facility Residents with *C. difficile*

Asymptomatic *C. difficile* colonization generally starts with ingestion of the *C. difficile* spores [1]. The spores survive the gastric acid and germinate into vegetative cells in the intestine. Vegetative *C. difficile* cells penetrate the mucus layer in the large intestine to adhere and colonize the intestinal epithelium. Even though *C. difficile* has been isolated from small intestine, it primarily colonizes the large intestine [1]. However, colonization with vegetative *C. difficile* cells usually requires a disruption of the normal intestinal microbiota [1]. Up to 70% of residents in a LTCF receive one or more courses of systemic antibiotics over a year which may contribute toward the disruption of the normal intestinal microbiota and place the residents of LTCF at higher risk for *C. difficile* colonization [34].

Rates of asymptomatic colonization with *C. difficile* range from 0% to 51% among residents of LTCF [1, 6, 35]. The rate of colonization by toxigenic strain of *C. difficile* strains has been shown to be 10 times higher in nursing home residents than in the community [6]. In addition, LTCF with known actual or recent CDI cases have been found to have a higher likelihood of having colonized residents as opposed to those without known *C. difficile* infection cases [6]. Preceding outbreaks of *C. difficile* infections may also increase the rate of colonization in a LTCF and can explain some of the variability in the reported rates of colonization among various studies [36]. In order to explore the epidemiology of *C. difficile* colonization in LTCF, Ziakas et al. conducted a meta-analysis consisting of nine studies (six from the USA, one from Canada, and two from Europe). The pooled colonization with toxigenic *C. difficile* was 14.8% (95% CI 7.6–24.0) among 1371 residents included in the meta-analysis [37]. However, colonization estimates were significantly higher in facilities with preceding CDI outbreaks as opposed to those without preceding outbreaks (30.1% vs. 6.5%, $p = 0.01$) [37].

It is important to realize that various studies have used different definitions of *C. difficile* colonization which may also impact the reported colonization rates [1, 38]. One of the definition that describes colonization well is suggested by Furuya-Kanamori et al. [1] They defined asymptomatic *C. difficile* colonization as "the absence of diarrhea (or if present, attributable to a cause other than CDI) without colonoscopic or histopathologic findings consistent with pseudomembranous colitis, and either the detection of *C. difficile* or the presence of *C. difficile* toxins." This definition takes into account that individuals who have colonization with *C. difficile* may also have diarrhea that is unrelated to the presence of *C. difficile* colonization. Consideration should be given to the possibility of other infectious, non-infectious, or iatrogenic (e.g., laxative overdose) causes of the diarrhea when differentiating between *C. difficile* colonization and infection particularly when nucleic acid amplification testing is used to identify *C. difficile*.

In general, several factors have been found to be associated with increased risk of *C. difficile* colonization. These include antibiotic exposure, hospitalization within the last 12 months, abdominal surgery, presence of nasogastric tubes, exposure to corticosteroids, history of *C. difficile* infection, chronic dialysis, use of proton-pump inhibitors or histamine H2 antagonists, chemotherapy, and presence of antibody against toxin B [1, 37]. One meta-analysis that looked specifically for factors associated with colonization in long-term care facilities found previous CDI, antibiotic use in the last 3 months, and hospitalization within the past 3 months to a year to be associated with *C. difficile* colonization [37]. The odds ratio for these three risk factors were 6.07 (95% CI 2.06–17.88), 3.68 (95% CI 2.04–6.62), and 2.11 (OR 2.11; 95% CI 1.08–4.13), respectively. No association of *C. difficile* colonization was found with age, gender, proton-pump inhibitor use, and comorbidities (including diabetes and urinary/fecal incontinence) in this analysis. Median length of stay in LTCF was also found to be similar between the *C. difficile* colonized and non-colonized residents. Additionally, the study reported no significant difference in the median length of stay between colonized and non-colonized residents. However, this study had several limitations and the authors of the study themselves cautioned against completely ruling out some of these factors like proton-pump inhibitor use as possible risk factors for *C. difficile* colonization in nursing homes given the presence of evidence outside the long-term care setting [39, 40].

Colonization rates in residents of LTCF may also depend on facility level characteristics [1]. Higher colonization rates have been seen in rehabilitation facilities [1, 38, 41]. One study showed 50% of spinal cord rehabilitation patients to be asymptomatically colonized with *C. difficile* [41]. This study also demonstrated that in comparison with non-colonized individuals, colonized individuals had higher rates of skin and environmental contamination along with longer length of stay. These factors may contribute to transmission within the facilities which can also impact the colonization rates. LTCF with higher proportion of shared occupancy rooms may also have the potential for higher colonization rates since living with roommates has been identified as a risk factor for CDI in long-term care setting [35, 42].

Transmission of *C. difficile* in Residents of Long-Term Care Facilities

Overall CDI incidence in any kind of setting depends on several factors that include transmission of *C. difficile* within the setting, use of antimicrobial drug, and underlying population health [7]. One of the studies estimated that hospitals have the highest transmission risk for CDI followed by the long-term care facilities and community [7]. According to this study estimate, a patient with CDI in a LTCF transmits *C. difficile* at a rate of 27% that for a comparable patient in the hospital. This transmission risk is much higher than the risk estimated for a patient in the community. A patient with CDI in the community transmits *C. difficile* to others at a rate of 0.1% that of a comparable patient in the hospital [7]. It has also been demonstrated that the risk of healthcare facility–acquired CDI is greater for those individuals who were admitted to the hospitals or skilled nursing facilities with higher than median prevalence of CDI [21]. Colonization of residents in LTCF with *C. difficile* also contributes to the transmission [37, 43–46]. Evidence suggest that *C. difficile* intestinal colonization may persist up to 6 months in some individuals, although fecal spore shedding becomes less common 5–6 weeks after treatment of CDI [1, 47]. It is also known that *C. difficile* may continue to persist on the skin beyond 4 weeks after therapy and on inanimate surfaces for as long as 5 months that might also contribute to transmission [48–50].

Durham et al. evaluated the impact of low-risk or high-risk antimicrobial agents for CDI on the incidence of CDI by using a drug risk ratio of 1–20 [7]. It was estimated that per unit increase in antimicrobial drug risk increases the CDI incidence by a factor of 33% in LTCF which is lower than what is expected in the hospital (160%) but higher than what is expected in community (6.4%). This suggests that magnitude of impact of specific antimicrobial drug use on CDI incidence also depends on the transmission rates within a facility.

Even though it has been shown that CDI transmission risk is much higher in hospitals as compared to the LTCF and the community, it is important to note that infection prevention and control programs and environmental cleaning and disinfection practices have been found to be more suboptimal in LTCF [7, 51–53]. Transmission in this setting is likely occurring by direct spread from the hands of the personnel, fomites, and the other objects in the environment. It may also be facilitated by the facts that the residents share spaces with others in the facility for sleeping, eating, and toileting along with attending social events together [11, 51]. During a CDI outbreak investigation in a 146-bed LTCF in the USA, *C. difficile* was isolated in environmental cultures throughout the institution including bed handrails, television remote control, doorway entrances, shower seat surface, wheelchair arms, toilet handrails, bedside table, sink surfaces, physical therapy grip handrail, dining room table top, and communal shower chairs [16]. This particular risk factor for transmission may get further amplified by the fact that 25–75% of antibiotic use in LTCF has been shown to be inappropriate and these facilities also lack well-developed antibiotic stewardship programs [34, 54, 55]. Majority of the antibiotic stewardship programs in the US LTCF are not meeting all seven CDC recommended core elements [55]. These factors represent some unique challenges related to preventing transmission of CDI in LTCF.

Risk Factors for *C. difficile* Infection and Colonization in Long-Term Care Facilities

Older adults, especially those residing in long-term care facilities, are at increased risk of acquiring *C. difficile* and developing severe disease associated with this infection [11]. Several factors have been identified that may contribute to this increased risk. Age-related changes in fecal flora and immunosenescence are among those contributing factors [15]. Lower gastric acidity, less *C. difficile* antibody production, and impaired *C. difficile* phagocytosis have been thought to play a role [56]. Environmental factors specific to long-term care setting, such as residents living in close proximity, shared rooms and toilet, and limited ability of the facility to properly isolate residents with infection, may also contribute toward *C. difficile* transmission, colonization, and infection [56]. In addition, antibiotic use, the presence of various underlying diseases, and the use of certain medications in the residents of long-term care facilities have been shown to be associated with CDI. These factors are further described in Table 2.1.

Table 2.1 Factors predisposing LTCF residents to higher risk for *C. difficile* colonization and infection

Category	Risk factors
Demographic factors	Increased age [11]
	White race [11]
Antibiotic use	Previous antibiotic use (especially in previous 3 months) [37]
	Use of antibiotics that has been identified as high risk for CDI acquisition [7, 15]
Use of other medications	Proton-pump inhibitor [57]
	Chemotherapy [11]
	H2 blockers [15]
	Use of steroid [58]
Systemic factors	Hypoalbuminemia [57]
	Renal failure/ESRD [10, 11]
	Pressure ulcers [11]
	Cirrhosis [11]
	Chronic obstructive pulmonary disease [11]
	Functional disability and cognitive impairment [56]
	Congestive heart failure [10]
	Cerebrovascular disease [10]
	≥3 comorbidities [9, 56]
Gastrointestinal factors	Fecal incontinence [11, 56]
	Prior *C difficile* infection [37]
Facility-related factors	Recent hospitalization (especially within previous 3 months to 1 year) [37]
	Frequent transition from LTCF to hospital [58]
	Residence in LTCF itself [7, 35]
Presence of devices	Presence of nasogastric tube [11, 15]
	Presence of gastrostomy tube [11, 15]
	Prior tracheostomy tube [11]

Mortality Associated with *C. difficile* Infection in Long-Term Care Facility Residents

In general, diarrhea is associated with a higher mortality in elderly as compared to the younger adults [9]. It has been shown that at least 30% of diarrheal deaths in elderly occur outside acute care setting, mainly in the nursing homes [9]. CDI is one of the predominant causes of infectious diarrhea in elderly residents living in nursing homes [9]. Based on active population- and laboratory-based surveillance across ten geographic areas in the USA, *C. difficile* was estimated to cause almost half a million infections and 29,000 deaths in 2011 [8]. The 30-day mortality rate was estimated to be 1.3% for community associated infections and 9.3% for healthcare-associated infections. However, studies that have looked specifically into mortality rates of CDI in nursing home residents have described higher mortality rates [10, 11].

A population-based retrospective cohort study focusing on US nursing homes by linking Medicare 5% random sample, Medicaid, and Minimum Data Set found the 30-day mortality after CDI episode to be 14.7% [10]. Mortality rates among CDI residents were consistently higher as compared to the non-CDI residents at 30-day (14.7% vs 4.3%, $p < 0.001$), 60-day (22.7% vs 7.5%, $p < 0.001$), 6-month (36.3% vs 18.3%, $p < 0.001$), and 1-year (48.2% vs 31.1%, $p < 0.001$) follow-up period. Total healthcare costs within 2 months following the first CDI episode were also significantly higher for those residents who had CDI as compared to those without CDI ($28,621 vs $13,644, $p < 0.001$). Overall, this study estimated 53,000 annual CDI cases in the residents of US long-term care facilities that were associated with 5500 deaths and $800 million in costs [10]. Another retrospective cohort study used US 2011 LTCF resident data from Minimum Data Set 3.0 linked to Medicare claims for examining the epidemiology of *C. difficile* in 2011 among LTCF residents >65 years old. Residents with CDI in this study also were found to have significantly higher mortality than those without CDI (24.7% vs 18.1%, $p = 0.001$). CDI was independently associated with mortality in multivariable analysis [11].

Conclusions

It is very clear that the epidemiology of CDI has changed significantly worldwide over the past two decades with increase in incidence and prevalence in all healthcare settings. This change is in part has been linked to the emergence of BI/NAP1/027 strain. This strain has been described as the most prevalent strain among inpatients admitted from LTCF and predominant strain in nursing home residents with CDI. It has also been implicated in several nursing home *C. difficile* infection outbreaks. *C. difficile* colonization rates in the residents of LTCF may also be higher after an outbreak. In general, the residents of long-term care facilities are at higher risk for *C. difficile* colonization and infection due to several different individual and facility specific risk factors. Mortality rates secondary to CDI are usually higher for LTCF residents. High prevalence of antibiotic misuse and lack of well-developed antimicrobial stewardship and infection prevention and control programs along with suboptimal environmental cleaning and disinfection practices can contribute toward more *C. difficile* transmission, colonization, and infections in LTCF. Efforts will need to be focused on addressing all modifiable individual and facility specific risk factors in order to decrease *C. difficile* incidence and prevalence in long-term care setting.

References

1. Furuya-Kanamori L, et al. Asymptomatic Clostridium difficile colonization: epidemiology and clinical implications. BMC Infect Dis. 2015;15:516.
2. Bartlett JG. Historical perspectives on studies of Clostridium difficile and C. difficile infection. Clin Infect Dis. 2008;46:S4–11.
3. Khanna S, Pardi DS. Clostridium difficile infection: management strategies for a difficult disease. Ther Adv Gastroenterol. 2014;7(2):72–86.
4. Migill SS, et al. Multistate point-prevalence survey of health care–associated infections. N Engl J Med. 2014;370:1198–208.
5. Centers for Disease Control and Prevention. Antibiotic resistance threats in the United States, 2013. CDC. https://www.cdc.gov/drugresistance/pdf/ar-threats-2013-508.pdf. Accessed 23 Apr 2013.

6. Arvand M, et al. High prevalence of *Clostridium difficile* colonization among nursing home residents in Hesse, Germany. PLoS One. 2012;7(1):e30183.
7. Durham DP, et al. Quantifying transmission of Clostridium difficile within and outside healthcare settings. Emerg Infect Dis. 2016;22(4):608–16.
8. Lessa FC, et al. Burden of *Clostridium difficile* infection in the United States. N Engl J Med. 2015;372:825–34.
9. Chopra T, et al. *Clostridium difficile* infection in long-term care facilities: a call to action for antimicrobial stewardship. Clin Infect Dis. 2015;60(S2):S72–6.
10. Yu H, et al. Burden of Clostridium difficile-associated disease among patients residing in nursing homes: a population-based cohort study. BMC Geriatr. 2016;16(1):193.
11. Ziakas PD, et al. Prevalence and impact of Clostridium difficile infection in elderly residents of long-term care facilities, 2011: a nationwide study. Medicine. 2016;95(31):e4187.
12. Freeman J, et al. The changing epidemiology of Clostridium difficile infections. Clin Microbiol Rev. 2010;23(3):529–49.
13. Zilberberg MD, et al. Increase in adult Clostridium difficile-related hospitalizations and case-fatality rate, United States, 2000–2005. Emerg Infect Dis. 2008;14(6):929–31.
14. Archbald-Pannone LR, et al. Clostridium difficile ribotype 027 is most prevalent among inpatients admitted from long-term care facilities. J Hosp Infect. 2014;88(4):218–21.
15. Simor AE, et al. Clostridium difficile in long-term-care facilities for the elderly. Infect Control Hosp Epidemiol. 2002;23(11):696–703.
16. Endres BT, et al. Environmental transmission of Clostridioides difficile ribotype 027 at a long-term care facility; an outbreak investigation guided by whole genome sequencing. Infect Control Hosp Epidemiol. 2018;39:1322–9.
17. Luk S, et al. High prevalence and frequent acquisition of Clostridium difficile ribotype 002 among nursing home residents in Hong Kong. Infect Control Hosp Epidemiol. 2018;39(7):782–7.
18. Rodriguez, et al. Longitudinal survey of *Clostridium difficile* presence and gut microbiota composition in a Belgian nursing home. BMC Microbiol. 2016;16:229.
19. Boone JH, et al. *Clostridium difficile* prevalence rates in a large healthcare system stratified according to patient population, age, gender, and specimen consistency. Eur J Clin Microbiol Infect Dis. 2012;31(7):1551–9.
20. CDC. Surveillance for community-associated Clostridium difficile--Connecticut, 2006. MMWR Morb Mortal Wkly Rep. 2008;57(13):340–3.
21. Joyce NR, et al. Effect of *Clostridium difficile* prevalence in hospitals and nursing homes on risk of infection. J Am Geriatr Soc. 2017;65:1527–34.
22. Dubberke ER, Olsen MA. Burden of *Clostridium difficile* on the healthcare system. Clin Infect Dis. 2012;55(Suppl 2):S88–92.

23. Shashank G, et al. Epidemiology of *Clostridium difficile*-associated disease (CDAD): a shift from hospital-acquired infection to long-term care facility-based infection. Dig Dis Sci. 2013;58:3407–12.
24. Pawar D, et al. Burden of *Clostridium difficile* infection in long-term care facilities in Monroe County. New York. Infect Control Hosp Epidemiol. 2012;33:1107–12.
25. Kim JH, et al. *Clostridium difficile* Infection in a long-term care facility: hospital-associated illness compared with long-term care–associated illness. Infect Control Hosp Epidemiol. 2011;32(7):656–60.
26. Zarowitz BJ, et al. Risk factors, clinical characteristics, and treatment differences between residents with and without nursing home- and non-nursing home-acquired Clostridium difficile infection. J Manag Care Spec Pharm. 2015;21(7):585–95.
27. Laffan AM, et al. Burden of Clostridium difficile-associated diarrhea in a long-term care facility. J Am Geriatr Soc. 2006;54(7):1068–73.
28. McDonald LC, et al. Recommendations for surveillance of Clostridium difficile-associated disease. Infect Control Hosp Epidemiol. 2007;28:140–5.
29. Centers for Disease Control and Prevention. Laboratory-identified Multidrug-Resistant Organism (MDRO) & *Clostridium difficile* infection (CDI) events for long-term care facilities. CDC. https://www.cdc.gov/nhsn/PDFs/LTC/LTCF-LabID-Event-Protocol_FINAL_8-24-12.pdf
30. Ponnada SP, et al. Acquisition of Clostridium difficile colonization and infection after transfer from a veterans affairs hospital to an affiliated long-term care facility. Infect Control Hosp Epidemiol. 2017;38:1070–6.
31. Guerrero DM, et al. Clostridium difficile infection in a Department of Veterans Affairs long-term care facility. Infect Control Hosp Epidemiol. 2011;32:513–5.
32. Hunter JC, et al. Burden of nursing home onset *Clostridium difficile* infection in the United States: estimates of incidence and patient outcomes. Open Forum Infect Dis. 2016;3:ofv196.
33. Mylotte JM, et al. Surveillance for *Clostridium difficile* infection in nursing homes. J Am Geriatr Soc. 2013;61:122–5.
34. Centers for Disease Control and Prevention. The core elements of antibiotic stewardship for nursing homes. Available at: http://www.cdc.gov/longtermcare/prevention/antibiotic-stewardship.html. Accessed 8 Jun 2019.
35. Jump RLP, Donskey CJ. Clostridium difficile in the long-term care facility: prevention and management. Curr Geriatr Rep. 2015;4(1):60–9.
36. Monique JT, et al. Understanding Clostridium difficile colonization. Clin Microbiol Rev. 2018;31:e00021–17.
37. Ziakas PD, et al. Asymptomatic carriers of toxigenic *C. difficile* in long-term care facilities: a meta-analysis of prevalence and risk factors. PLoS One. 2015;10(2):e0117195.
38. Schaffler H, Breitruck A. *Clostridium difficile* – from colonization to infection. Front Microbiol. 2018;9:646.

39. Loo VG, et al. Host and pathogen factors for *Clostridium difficile* infection and colonization. N Engl J Med. 2011;365:1693–703.
40. Jump RL, et al. Vegetative *Clostridium difficile* survives in room air on moist surfaces and in gastric contents with reduced acidity: a potential mechanism to explain the association between proton pump inhibitors and C. difficile-associated diarrhea? Antimicrob Agents Chemother. 2007;51(8):2883–7.
41. Dumford DM, et al. Epidemiology of *Clostridium difficile* and vancomycin-resistant Enterococcus colonization in patients on a spinal cord injury unit. J Spinal Cord Med. 2011;34(1):22–7.
42. Vesteinsdottir I, et al. Risk factors for Clostridium difficile toxin-positive diarrhea: a population-based prospective case-control study. Eur J Clin Microbiol Infect Dis. 2012;31(10):2601–10.
43. Donskey CJ, et al. Transmission of *Clostridium difficile* from asymptomatically colonized or infected long-term care facility residents. Infect Control Hosp Epidemiol. 2018;39(8):909–16.
44. Riggs MM, et al. Asymptomatic carriers are a potential source for transmission of epidemic and nonepidemic *Clostridium difficile* strains among long-term care facility residents. Clin Infect Dis. 2007;45(8):992–8.
45. Galdys AL, et al. Asymptomatic *Clostridium difficile* colonization as a reservoir for Clostridium difficile infection. Expert Rev Anti-Infect Ther. 2014;12:967–80.
46. Curry SR, et al. Use of multilocus variable number of tandem repeats analysis genotyping to determine the role of asymptomatic carriers in *Clostridium difficile* transmission. Clin Infect Dis. 2013;57:1094–102.
47. Jinno S, et al. Potential for transmission of *Clostridium difficile* by asymptomatic acute care patients and long-term care facility residents with prior *C. difficile* infection. Infect Control Hosp Epidemiol. 2012;33(6):638–9.
48. Rodriguez C, et al. Clostridium difficile infection in elderly nursing home residents. Anaerobe. 2014;30:184–7.
49. Sethi AK, et al. Persistence of skin contamination and environmental shedding of Clostridium difficile during and after treatment of *C. difficile* infection. Infect Control Hosp Epidemiol. 2010;31:21–7.
50. Kramer A, et al. How long do nosocomial pathogens persist on inanimate surfaces? A systematic review. BMC Infect Dis. 2006;6:130.
51. Quinn LK, et al. Infection control policies and practices for Iowa long-term care facility residents with Clostridium difficile infection. Infect Control Hosp Epidemiol. 2007;28(11):1228–32.
52. Ashraf MS, et al. Environmental cleaning and disinfection policies, protocols and practices: a survey of 27 long-term care facilities. Presented at SHEA 2018; April 18–20, 2018; Portland, OR. Abstract 10159 (Poster 214) Available at: https://shea.confex.com/shea/2018/meetingapp.cgi/Paper/10159. Accessed 9 June 2019.
53. Nailon RE, et al. Impact of an audit and feedback program on environmental cleaning and disinfection in critical access hospitals and long-

term care facilities. Presented at APIC 2018; June 13–15; Minneapolis, MN: American Journal of Infection Control, Volume 46, Issue 6, S29.

54. Van Schooneveld T. Survey of antimicrobial stewardship practices in Nebraska long-term care facilities. Infect Control Hosp Epidemiol. 2011;32(7):732–4.

55. Lodhi HT, et al. Abstract 1838. Digging deeper: a closer look at core elements of antibiotic stewardship for long-term care facilities. Open Forum Infect Dis. 2018;5(Suppl 1):S524.

56. Simor AE. Diagnosis, management, and prevention of *Clostridium difficile* infection in long-term care facilities: a review. J Am Geriatr Soc. 2010;58:1556–64.

57. Al-Tureihi FI, et al. Albumin, length of stay, and proton pump inhibitors: key factors in Clostridium difficile-associated disease in nursing home patients. J Am Med Dir Assoc. 2005;6(2):105–8.

58. Haran JP, et al. Medication exposure and risk of recurrent Clostridium difficile infection in community-dwelling older people and nursing home residents. J Am Geriatr Soc. 2018;66(2):333–8.

Role of Asymptomatic Carriers in Long-Term Care Facility *Clostridioides* (*Clostridium*) *difficile* Transmission

3

Ravina Kullar and Ellie J. C. Goldstein

Introduction

Clostridioides (*Clostridium*) *difficile* remains the leading cause of healthcare-associated diarrhea and is responsible for 500,000 illnesses and up to 30,000 deaths annually in the United States [1–4]. The annual cost of treatment associated with CDI ranges from $1.9 to $7.0 billion [5]. Over the last two decades, there has been a worldwide increase in the incidence and severity of CDI, with the Centers for Disease Control and Prevention (CDC) designating *C. difficile* as an urgent threat [1, 6]. Its clinical manifestations range from asymptomatic carriage to severe forms of fulminant colitis and death [7]. Major risk factors for CDI are well known and include exposure to antibiotics, usage of proton-pump inhibitors (PPIs), prior and prolonged hospitalizations, chemotherapy, immunocompromised status, multiple comorbidities, hypoalbuminemia,

R. Kullar
Expert Stewardship Inc., Newport Beach, CA, USA

E. J. C. Goldstein (✉)
Infectious Diseases Division, Providence St Johns' Health Center, RM Alden Research Laboratory, Santa Monica, CA, USA

© Springer Nature Switzerland AG 2020   25
T. Chopra (ed.), *Clostridium Difficile Infection in Long-Term Care Facilities*, https://doi.org/10.1007/978-3-030-29772-5_3

renal insufficiency, use of nasogastric tubes, gastrointestinal surgeries, and advanced age [8–11].

Healthcare-related infections have declined significantly in US hospitals from 2011 to 2015 (2011: 452 [4.0%; 95% confidence interval (CI), 3.7–4.4] vs. 394 patients [3.2%; 95% CI 2.9–3.5] ($P < 0.001$)), according to a recent point-prevalence survey [12]. Most of these reductions occurred in surgical site and urinary tract infections. However, the prevalence of healthcare-related pneumonia and *C. difficile* did not decline during the study period, highlighting that progress is still needed in prevention strategies for these infections. Based on recent data from the CDC's Emerging Infections Program (EIP), the incidence of CDI is the highest among those aged ≥65 years (627.7). Of the total estimated 453,000 incident cases, 293,300 (64.7%) were healthcare-associated, of which 37% were hospital-onset, and 36% had their onset in long-term care facilities (LTCFs) [13]. Further, many patients diagnosed with CDI in hospitals are typically discharged to LTCFs [14].

In the United States, 15,600 LTCFs provide care to >3 million people each year [15]. The number of older adults requiring long-term care services is anticipated to increase to 19 million by 2050 [16]. By 2050, there will be >80 million older persons, over twice their number in 2000. People ≥65 represented 14.1% of the population in the year 2013 but are expected to grow to be >20% of the population by 2050 [17]. Accordingly, distinct to LTCFs, a high percentage of residents are *C. difficile* colonized, with rates of asymptomatic colonization among LTCF residents ranging from 5% to 51% (compared to 1–3% among the general population) [18–21]. Determining the significance that these asymptomatic carriers play in transmitting CDI is important to determine the effectiveness of facility-based measures to control infection. Further, toxin-targeting treatments, such as vaccines and monoclonal antibodies, may protect against CDI but are unlikely to prevent asymptomatic colonization with *C. difficile* [22]. Therefore, this chapter will focus on literature discussing the role of asymptomatic carriers in LTCFs in CDI transmission.

Definition and Detection of *C. difficile* Colonization

Asymptomatic *C. difficile* colonization refers to the shedding of *C. difficile* in stool but without diarrhea or other clinical symptoms [11]. Shim et al. revealed that asymptomatic *C. difficile* colonized patients in the acute care setting may be protected from progression to infection since they can mount a humoral immune response to clostridial toxins [23]. However, asymptomatic *C. difficile* colonized patients may act as an infection reservoir, transmitting *C. difficile* onto other patients [19, 24]. Although these asymptomatic patients shed spores into the environment to a lesser extent than CDI patients, by outnumbering the CDI patients, they can still play a crucial role in transmission of the disease [19, 25].

The Infectious Diseases Society of America (IDSA)/Society for Healthcare Epidemiology of America (SHEA) 2018 CDI guidelines recommend diagnostic testing only in those patients with unexplained and new-onset ≥3 unformed stools in 24 hours, with nucleic acid amplification tests (NAAT) alone or a multistep algorithm recommended for testing (i.e., glutamate dehydrogenase (GDH) plus toxin; GDH plus toxin, arbitrated by NAAT; or NAAT plus toxin). Screening for asymptomatic carriage and placing asymptomatic carriers on contact precautions are not recommended unless there is an outbreak [11]. However, given that CDI has not declined over the years, the shift in healthcare delivery to transitions of care with "sharing of patients," and increased risk for CDI in LTCFs, rethinking these recommendations is warranted. Currently, an optimal diagnostic method that can accurately differentiate CDI compared to colonization does not exist. Literature in asymptomatically colonized patients varies significantly in patient inclusion criteria, tested material, and applied diagnostic and gold standard tests. For instance, various studies only test rectal swabs or use a combination of stool samples and rectal swabs [25–29]. Guerrero et al. revealed that asymptomatic carriers in LTCFs have lower numbers of *C. difficile* in their rectal swab compared to CDI patients, suggesting that stool samples are preferred [25]. Additionally, various diagnostic screening tests have been used to detect *C. difficile*, frequently divided into assays to recognize toxigenic or nontoxigenic strains [11, 30]. A comparison of different diagnostic tests with a reference method to detect asymptomatic *C. difficile* colonization is warranted.

Asymptomatic Carriage and *C. difficile* Transmission in LTCFs

While several studies have focused on the pathogenesis and the development of CDI, the role of asymptomatic *C. difficile* colonization in LTCFs and its progression to CDI in LTCFs is still not clear. Donskey et al. recently conducted a prospective cohort study in a Veterans Affairs hospital and its affiliated LTCF to determine the role of LTCF patients with CDI or asymptomatic carriage in the transmission of toxigenic *C. difficile* strains [31]. Of the 201 LTCF residents screened, 29 (14.4%) were classified as asymptomatic carriers of toxigenic *C. difficile* based on every other week perirectal screening, and 37.9% were transferred to the hospital at least once. Overall, 37 healthcare-associated CDI cases were reported, including 26 that were acquired in the hospital and 11 that were acquired in the LTCF. Of the 37 CDI cases, seven (18.9%) were linked to LTCF residents with LTCF-associated CDI or asymptomatic carriage. Of the seven transmissions linked to LTCF residents, five (71.4%) were linked to asymptomatic carriers versus two (28.6%) to CDI cases, and all involved transmission of epidemic BI/NAP1/027strains. Of note, all four of the carriers linked to transmission had a relatively high burden of carriage (i.e., >25 colonies/perirectal swab), suggesting that such carriers may present the greatest risk for transmission. These results indicate that LTCF residents with asymptomatic carriage of *C. difficile* or CDI may contribute substantially to transmission.

In an outbreak setting, Riggs and colleagues prospectively examined the prevalence of asymptomatic carriage of NAP1 and non-epidemic toxigenic *C. difficile* strains in LTCF patients and evaluated the frequency of environmental and skin contamination [19]. Over a 3-month period, they observed 73 LTCF residents, with 35 (51%) being asymptomatic carriers and 13 (37%) of these 35 patients carrying epidemic NAP1 strains. Residents with asymptomatic carriage outnumbered those with CDI by a factor of 7 to 1. Compared with noncarriers, asymptomatic carriers had higher percentages of skin (61% vs. 19%; $P = 0.001$) and environmental contamination (59% vs. 24%; $P = 0.004$). The combination of prior *C. difficile*-associated disease and previous antibiotic use was predictive of asymptomatic carriage. These findings suggest that asymptomatic carriers have the potential to contribute to the transmission of epidemic and nonepidemic *C. difficile* infection in LTCFs. However, it is important to keep in mind that asymptomatic carriage leading to CDI transmission contributes to a minority of overall transmission.

Garg et al. studied the epidemiological changing trends of patients presenting with *Clostridium-difficile*-associated diarrhea (CDAD) admitted to an acute-care hospital and evaluated the factors contributing to this shift in epidemiology [32]. Two-hundred and fifty-six toxin-positive CDAD patients were included, with 53 (20.6%) patients having hospital-acquired CDAD. Patients from LTCFs ($N = 119$, 46.1%) and the community (86 patients, 33.3%) comprised 79.4% of patients. Most LTCF patients ($n = 101$, 84.8%) had non-diarrheal symptoms as their presenting complaint as compared to only 61 patients from the community (70.9%) ($P < 0.05$). These results suggest that CDAD originated primarily in patients from LTCFs (46.1%), with a majority of these patients being asymptomatic.

A cohort study was performed to determine the association of clinical variables with *C. difficile* colonization in patients admitted to a geriatric unit in Germany [33]. At admission, 43 (16.4%) patients tested positive for toxin B by PCR. Seven (16.3%) of these colonized patients developed clinical CDI during hospital stay. Overall, seven out of eight (87.5%) CDI patients had been colonized at admission. Risk factors of colonization with *C. difficile* were a history of CDI and previous antibiotic treatment and hospital stays. This study shows the impact that colonization can have on the subsequent development of symptomatic CDI.

A systematic review and meta-analysis evaluated the epidemiology of *C. difficile* colonization in LTCFs to determine the subsequent risk of infection [34]. Nine studies were included and comprised 1371 patients. Ziakas et al. found that 14.8% (95% CI 7.6–24.0%) of LTCF residents were asymptomatic carriers of toxigenic *C. difficile*. Colonization rates were significantly higher in facilities with prior CDI outbreak (30.1% vs. 6.5%, $P = 0.01$). Patient history of CDI (OR 6.07; 95% CI 2.06–17.88), prior hospitalization (OR 2.11; 95% CI 1.08–4.13), and antimicrobial use within previous 3 months (OR 3.68; 95% CI 2.04–6.62) were associated with colonization. Further, a simulation analysis revealed that on average two new *C. difficile* carriers will occur in LTCFs for every three individuals colonized at admission. These findings suggest that infection prevention measures should potentially extend to colonized LTCF residents harboring toxigenic strains.

Impact of Carriage in the Non-LTCF Setting

Several studies have suggested that asymptomatic carriers in the non-LTCF setting may also be a source of transmission [35–37]. In a long-term acute care hospital (LTACH) in Los Angeles, 36 patients were monitored for a 1-month period while they were receiving treatment [38]. Four patients tested antigen (+) with *C. difficile* upon admission; two had unsuspected, active disease; and two were carriers and did not experience any symptoms. During the individual courses of treatment of the patients, 55.5% of the patients being followed had symptoms of diarrhea, whereas five patients (13.8%) were eventually diagnosed with CDI. In a tertiary care hospital, Curry and colleagues used multilocus variable number of tandem repeats analysis (MLVA) to determine the genetic relationships between isolates from asymptomatic carriers and patients with healthcare-associated CDI [35]. Of 3006 patients screened, 314 (10.4%) were positive for toxigenic *C. difficile*. Of 56 incident cases of CDI classified as healthcare associated, 17 (30%) cases were associated with CDI patients, whereas 16 (29%) cases were associated with carriers. Further, in a quasi-experimental study conducted in a Canadian hospital, Longtin et al. demonstrated that a hospital-based intervention involving detection and isolation of *C. difficile* carriers was associated with a significant ($P < 0.001$) decrease in the incidence of healthcare-associated CDI [36]. Moreover, a systematic review and meta-analysis revealed that in the acute-care setting, >8% of admitted patients are carriers of toxinogenic *C. difficile* with an almost six times higher risk of infection [39]. Whole genome sequencing of *C. difficile* strains has also confirmed that transmission attributed to symptomatic patients accounts only for a minority of CDI acquisitions and that asymptomatic carriers contribute to the chain of transmission [40]. These studies highlight the impact of colonization in CDI epidemiology and stress the importance of preventive measures toward colonized patients.

Conclusion

Patients in LTCFs carry an increased susceptibility to acquiring CDI due to environmental factors, such as residence in close, shared quarters, communal toilet facilities, and limited ability to isolate infected residents. In addition, this population carries intrinsic factors such as advanced age, immune and physiologic senescence, and multiple comorbid conditions that contribute to their increased risk for CDI [41]. In fact, ~60% of LTCF residents are >80 years old and have a median length of stay of 33 days (interquartile range 19–90 days) [34]. Many of these patients are also placed on multiple courses of antibiotics, which is directly linked to CDI. To help curb CDI and antimicrobial resistance (AMR), the Centers for Medicare & Medicaid Services (CMS) mandated LTCFs to have antimicrobial stewardship programs (ASPs) in place as of 28 November 2017 [42]. LTCFs are often underfunded, understaffed, and overwhelmed with patients, making the implementation of ASPs difficult [43]. However, restricting inappropriate antimicrobial usage in addition to optimizing infection control measures in this setting needs to be made a priority [38]. Utilizing resources from the local public health department and a neighboring acute-care hospital has been shown to aid with the implementation of antimicrobial stewardship initiatives in this setting [44].

Literature discussing the role that asymptomatic carriers play in LTCF CDI transmission is sparse. It has not been conclusively determined in what way asymptomatic carriage in LTCFs affects the risk of a symptomatic CDI disease nor to what degree it plays a role in the spreading of the pathogen. Albeit not studied in the LTCF setting, positive screening for toxigenic *C. difficile* carriage at admission has been shown to provide a high predictive value for subsequent development of a symptomatic CDI [35, 45]. Knowing a patient's carrier status at admission could be beneficial to an LTCF, and in positive cases, it would offer options on how to manage the scenario: providing efficient hygiene management of these patients (i.e., infection prevention procedures) would curtail the spread of the pathogen, and the number of subsequent CDI cases could be reduced. We recommend a risk-adapted algorithm in asymptomatic carriers in the LTCF setting, including, upon admission, screening high-risk patients with prior episodes of CDI, previous hospitalization, and prior antibiotic treatment. It is important to keep in mind that LTCFs are the long-term residence of many patients and the need to isolate a patient due to asymptomatic CDI must be balanced with providing a home-like environment. Further studies evaluating the clinical consequences of asymptomatic *C. difficile* colonization are needed.

Conflicts of Interest RK has no conflicts of interest. EJCG Advisory boards: Merck & Co, Bayer Pharmaceuticals, Bio-K+, Cutis Pharmaceuticals, Sanofi-Aventis, Summit Corp. PLC, Kindred Healthcare Corp., Daiichi Sankyo, Paratek Pharma, and Shionogi Inc.; Speakers' bureau: Bayer Inc., Merck & Co, Medicines Co., and Allergan Inc.; Research grants: Bayer Inc., Cutis Pharmaceuticals, Entasis Therapeutics, Merck & Co, Micromyx LLC, Paratek Pharmaceuticals, Spero Therapeutics, and Tetraphase Therapeutics.

References

1. Centers for Disease Control and Prevention. Threat report 2013. Antimicrobial Resistance. Available at: http://www.cdc.gov/drugresistance/threat-report-2013/index.html. Accessed 15 Oct 2018.
2. Lessa FC, Mu Y, Bamberg WM, et al. Burden of Clostridium difficile infection in the United States. N Engl J Med. 2015;372:825–34.

3. Hall AJ, Curns AT, McDonald LC, et al. The roles of Clostridium difficile and norovirus among gastroenteritis-associated deaths in the United States, 1999–2007. Clin Infect Dis. 2012;55:216–23.
4. Lawson PA, Citron DM, Tyrrell KL, et al. Reclassification of Clostridium difficile as Clostridioides difficile (Hall and O'Toole 1935) Prevot 1938. Anaerobe. 2016;40:95–9.
5. Zhang S, Palazuelos-Munoz S, Balsells EM, et al. Cost of hospital management of Clostridium difficile infection in United States-a meta-analysis and modelling study. BMC Infect Dis. 2016;16:447.
6. Khanna S, Pardi DS. The growing incidence and severity of Clostridium difficile infection in inpatient and outpatient settings. Expert Rev Gastroenterol Hepatol. 2010;4:409–16.
7. DiDiodato G, McArthur L. Evaluating the effectiveness of an antimicrobial stewardship program on reducing the incidence rate of healthcare-associated Clostridium difficile infection: a non-randomized, stepped wedge, single-site, observational study. PLoS One. 2016;11:e0157671.
8. Loo VG, Bourgault AM, Poirier L, et al. Host and pathogen factors for Clostridium difficile infection and colonization. N Engl J Med. 2011;365:1693–703.
9. McDonald LC, Owings M, Jernigan DB. Clostridium difficile infection in patients discharged from US short-stay hospitals, 1996–2003. Emerg Infect Dis. 2006;12:409–15.
10. Thibault A, Miller MA, Gaese C. Risk factors for the development of Clostridium difficile-associated diarrhea during a hospital outbreak. Infect Control Hosp Epidemiol. 1991;12:345–8.
11. McDonald LC, Gerding DN, Johnson S, et al. Clinical practice guidelines for Clostridium difficile infection in adults and children: 2017 update by the Infectious Diseases Society of America (IDSA) and Society for Healthcare Epidemiology of America (SHEA). Clin Infect Dis. 2018;66:987–94.
12. Magill SS, O'Leary E, Janelle SJ, et al. Changes in prevalence of health care-associated infections in U.S. hospitals. N Engl J Med. 2018;379:1732–44.
13. Centers for Disease Control and Prevention. Emerging infections program—healthcare-associated infections projects. 2015. Available at: http://www.cdc.gov/hai/eip/index.html. Accessed 15 Oct 2018.
14. Kazakova SV, Ware K, Baughman B, et al. A hospital outbreak of diarrhea due to an emerging epidemic strain of Clostridium difficile. Arch Intern Med. 2006;166:2518–24.
15. Centers for Medicare and Medicaid Services. CMS survey and certification group 2016/2017 nursing home action plan. Available at: https://www.cms.gov/Medicare/Provider-Enrollment-and-Certification/CertificationandComplianc/Downloads/2016-2017-Nursing-Home-Action-Plan.pdf. Accessed 3 Nov 2018.

16. Department of Health and Human Services, Office of the Assistant Secretary for Planning and Evaluation. The future supply of long-term care workers in relation to the aging baby boom generation: report to Congress [Internet]. Washington, DC: HHS; 2003. Available from: http://aspe.hhs.gov/daltcp/reports/ltcwork.htm. Accessed 3 Nov 2018.

17. Census Bureau. 2012 national population projections: summary tables: Table 4: projections of the population by sex, race, and Hispanic origin for the United States: 2015 to 2060 [Internet]. Washington, DC: Census Bureau. Available from: http://www.census.gov/population/projections/data/national/2012/summarytables.html. Accessed 3 Nov 2018.

18. Bender BS, Bennett R, Laughon BE, et al. Is Clostridium difficile endemic in chronic-care facilities? Lancet. 1986;2:11–3.

19. Riggs MM, Sethi AK, Zabarsky TF, et al. Asymptomatic carriers are a potential source for transmission of epidemic and nonepidemic Clostridium difficile strains among long-term care facility residents. Clin Infect Dis. 2007;45:992–8.

20. Rea MC, O'Sullivan O, Shanahan F, et al. Clostridium difficile carriage in elderly subjects and associated changes in the intestinal microbiota. J Clin Microbiol. 2012;50:867–75.

21. Arvand M, Moser V, Schwehn C, et al. High prevalence of Clostridium difficile colonization among nursing home residents in Hesse, Germany. PLoS One. 2012;7:e30183.

22. Gerding DN, Johnson S. Management of Clostridium difficile infection: thinking inside and outside the box. Clin Infect Dis. 2010;51:1306–13.

23. Shim JK, Johnson S, Samore MH, et al. Primary symptomless colonisation by Clostridium difficile and decreased risk of subsequent diarrhoea. Lancet. 1998;351:633–6.

24. McFarland LV, Mulligan ME, Kwok RY, et al. Nosocomial acquisition of Clostridium difficile infection. N Engl J Med. 1989;320:204–10.

25. Guerrero DM, Becker JC, Eckstein EC, et al. Asymptomatic carriage of toxigenic Clostridium difficile by hospitalized patients. J Hosp Infect. 2013;85:155–8.

26. Marciniak C, Chen D, Stein AC, et al. Prevalence of Clostridium difficile colonization at admission to rehabilitation. Arch Phys Med Rehabil. 2006;87:1086–90.

27. Alasmari F, Seiler SM, Hink T, et al. Prevalence and risk factors for asymptomatic Clostridium difficile carriage. Clin Infect Dis. 2014;59:216–22.

28. Sall O, Johansson K, Noren T. Low colonization rates of Clostridium difficile among patients and healthcare workers at Orebro University Hospital in Sweden. APMIS. 2015;123:240–4.

29. Samore MH, DeGirolami PC, Tlucko A, et al. Clostridium difficile colonization and diarrhea at a tertiary care hospital. Clin Infect Dis. 1994;18:181–7.

30. Crobach MJ, Planche T, Eckert C, et al. European Society of Clinical Microbiology and Infectious Diseases: update of the diagnostic guidance document for Clostridium difficile infection. Clin Microbiol Infect. 2016;22(Suppl 4):S63–81.
31. Donskey CJ, Sunkesula VCK, Stone ND, et al. Transmission of Clostridium difficile from asymptomatically colonized or infected long-term care facility residents. Infect Control Hosp Epidemiol. 2018;39:909–16.
32. Garg S, Mirza YR, Girotra M, et al. Epidemiology of Clostridium difficile-associated disease (CDAD): a shift from hospital-acquired infection to long-term care facility-based infection. Dig Dis Sci. 2013;58:3407–12.
33. Nissle K, Kopf D, Rosler A. Asymptomatic and yet C. difficile-toxin positive? Prevalence and risk factors of carriers of toxigenic Clostridium difficile among geriatric in-patients. BMC Geriatr. 2016;16:185.
34. Ziakas PD, Zacharioudakis IM, Zervou FN, et al. Asymptomatic carriers of toxigenic C. difficile in long-term care facilities: a meta-analysis of prevalence and risk factors. PLoS One. 2015;10:e0117195.
35. Curry SR, Muto CA, Schlackman JL, et al. Use of multilocus variable number of tandem repeats analysis genotyping to determine the role of asymptomatic carriers in Clostridium difficile transmission. Clin Infect Dis. 2013;57:1094–102.
36. Longtin Y, Paquet-Bolduc B, Gilca R, et al. Effect of detecting and isolating Clostridium difficile carriers at hospital admission on the incidence of C difficile infections: a quasi-experimental controlled study. JAMA Intern Med. 2016;176:796–804.
37. Blixt T, Gradel KO, Homann C, et al. Asymptomatic carriers contribute to nosocomial Clostridium difficile infection: a cohort study of 4508 patients. Gastroenterology. 2017;152:1031–41 e2.
38. Goldstein EJ, Polonsky J, Touzani M, et al. C. difficile infection (CDI) in a long-term acute care facility (LTAC). Anaerobe. 2009;15:241–3.
39. Zacharioudakis IM, Zervou FN, Pliakos EE, et al. Colonization with toxinogenic C. difficile upon hospital admission, and risk of infection: a systematic review and meta-analysis. Am J Gastroenterol. 2015;110:381–90.. quiz 91
40. Didelot X, Eyre DW, Cule M, et al. Microevolutionary analysis of Clostridium difficile genomes to investigate transmission. Genome Biol. 2012;13:R118.
41. Simor AE. Diagnosis, management, and prevention of Clostridium difficile infection in long-term care facilities: a review. J Am Geriatr Soc. 2010;58:1556–64.
42. Centers for Medicare & Medicaid Services. CMS issues proposed rule that prohibits discrimination, reduces hospital-acquired conditions, and promotes antibiotic stewardship in hospitals. Available at: https://www.

cms.gov/Newsroom/MediaReleaseDatabase/Fact-sheets/2016-Fact-sheets-items/2016-06-13.html. Accessed 3 Nov 2018.

43. Nicolle LE, Bentley DW, Garibaldi R, et al. Antimicrobial use in long-term-care facilities. SHEA Long-Term-Care Committee. Infect Control Hosp Epidemiol. 2000;21:537–45.

44. Kullar R, Yang H, Grein J, et al. A roadmap to implementing antimicrobial stewardship principles in long-term care facilities (LTCFs): collaboration between an acute-care hospital and LTCFs. Clin Infect Dis. 2018;66:1304–12.

45. Starr JM, Martin H, McCoubrey J, et al. Risk factors for Clostridium difficile colonisation and toxin production. Age Ageing. 2003;32:657–60.

Clostridium difficile (Clostridioides difficile) Infection Surveillance in Long-Term Care Facilities

4

Amar Krishna and Justin Oring

Surveillance involves systematic collection, consolidation, and analysis of data on healthcare-associated infections (HAIs) [1]. Every long-term care facility (LTCF) should have a system for ongoing collection of data on HAIs including *Clostridium* (*Clostridioides*) *difficile* infection (CDI). LTCFs should assign an Infection Control Professional (ICP) who in turn is responsible for conducting HAI surveillance and directing infection control activities in the LTCF. The ICP is commonly a registered nurse who has specific training in infection control. The ICP should perform surveillance at least on a weekly basis, and the information thus collected including HAI rates should then be used to guide infection control activities and plan educational programs and shared with relevant committees/personnel/public health authorities [1]. The ICP should be provided with support and resources by the LTCF administration to carry out surveillance and effectively direct the infection control program at the LTCF [1].

CDI surveillance in LTCFs will help determine the burden of CDI in LTCF [2]. Analyzing the infection rates detected by surveil-

A. Krishna (✉) · J. Oring
Detroit Medical Center/Wayne State University, Detroit, MI, USA
e-mail: akrishn@med.wayne.edu

© Springer Nature Switzerland AG 2020
T. Chopra (ed.), *Clostridium Difficile Infection in Long-Term Care Facilities*, https://doi.org/10.1007/978-3-030-29772-5_4

lance will help determine infection trends and detect outbreaks [1, 2]. It will also help determine the effectiveness of infection control and antibiotic stewardship interventions administered to control spread of *Clostridium* (*Clostridioides*) *difficile* in an LTCF [1, 2]. When a facility notices increases in CDI incidence rates from a baseline rate or if the incidence is higher than in comparable institutions, then surveillance data should be stratified by location or clinical service to identify particular patient populations where infection control efforts can be targeted [3]. In addition to performing CDI surveillance, LTCFs should also collect and analyze data on process measures relevant to CDI infection control such as monitoring hand hygiene and contact isolation compliance [1]. These data might help explain changes in CDI rates in the LTCF or a specific unit in an LTCF and will help guide infection control efforts.

Currently, reporting of CDI events via National Healthcare Safety Network (NHSN) is a mandatory requirement for acute care hospitals participating in Centers for Medicare & Medicaid Services (CMS) hospital inpatient quality reporting (IQR) program and is used to determine payment incentives [4]. However, reporting of CDI events by LTCFs to CMS is currently voluntary [4]. A recent study showed that during January 2013 to December 2015, only 147 of the approximately 15,600 nursing homes/LTCFs reportedly operating in the United States completed at least 1 month of CDI surveillance. The number of nursing homes reporting consistently (≥ 6 months) was even less. Not-for-profit nursing homes, nursing homes affiliated with a multifacility chain, and nursing homes attached to hospitals were more likely to perform CDI surveillance [4].

Some of the barriers to voluntary reporting in LTCFs include limited time and resources, competing priorities, high staff turnover, limitations in IT (information technology) infrastructure, and inability to maximize benefit of surveillance due to limited interpretation capacity [5]. Collaboration with external partners/programs can drive surveillance activities in LTCFs as it maintains accountability and engagement, provides a forum to share experiences, and provides resources to translate surveillance data to prevention actions [5].

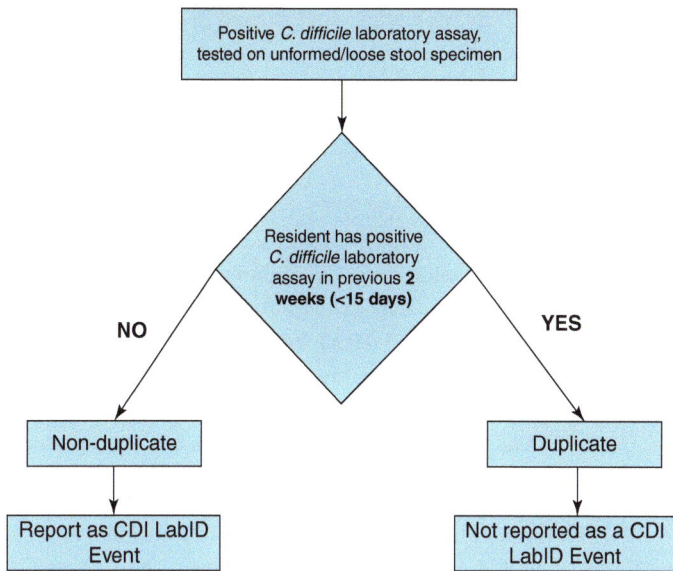

Fig. 4.1 *C. difficile* test result algorithm for laboratory-identified (LabID) events. *Notes*: (1) LabID event reporting is based on specimens collected by the LTCF during the care of the resident and specimens collected in an ED or OP (e.g., physician's office) during the current admission. Laboratory results obtained prior to the resident's admission to the LTCF or during an admission in another healthcare facility are excluded. (2) Day of specimen collection equals day one of the specimen count. (This figure was adapted from Ref. [2])

NHSN uses laboratory-identified (LabID) event reporting for CDI surveillance in both acute care hospitals and nursing home/ LTCFs [2]. This method uses positive lab tests to tract CDI rates without the need for clinical evaluation of patient for signs and symptoms and therefore is less labor intensive [2]. The three definitions commonly used by NHSN for CDI surveillance in LTCFs further elaborated in Fig. 4.1 are as follows:

- *C. difficile* **positive laboratory assay:** Unformed/loose stool that tests positive for *C. difficile* toxin A and/or B (includes molecular assays [PCR] and/or toxin assays) or a toxin-producing *C. difficile* organism detected in an unformed/loose stool sample by culture or other laboratory means [2].

- **CDI LabID event:** Non-duplicate *C. difficile* positive laboratory assay obtained while a resident is receiving care from the long-term care facility or a non-duplicate positive result obtained from an emergency department or outpatient setting, during a resident's current admission in LTCF (specifically, no change in current admission date in LTCF). Laboratory results obtained before a resident's admission to LTCF or during admission in another facility are excluded from CDI reporting [2].
- **Duplicate *C. difficile* positive laboratory assay:** Any *C. difficile* positive laboratory assay from the same resident following a previous *C. difficile* positive laboratory assay within the past 2 weeks (<15 days). Duplicate assays are not reported to NHSN [2].

NHSN further classifies CDI LabID event as incident or recurrent based on the specimen collection date for the current CDI event and the specimen collection date (if any) of a previous CDI LabID event [2]:

- **Incident CDI** is defined as either the first CDI LabID event for an individual resident in the facility or a CDI event reported >56 days (8 weeks) after the individuals previous CDI event.
- **Recurrent CDI** is defined as any CDI LabID event >14 days (2 weeks) and <57 days (8 weeks) after the most recent CDI event reported for an individual resident.

All incident and recurrent CDI LabID events are further categorized into community onset and LTCF onset based on the date of current admission to the facility and date specimen collected (event date) [2]. Such classification will help determine the setting (LTCF or community) where CDI was likely acquired.

- **Community onset:** Date specimen collected ≤3 calendar days after date of current admission to the facility (specifically, day 1, 2, or 3 of admission)
- **LTCF onset:** Date specimen collected >3 calendar days after date of current admission to the facility (specifically, on or after day 4)

It is also important to determine recent exposure to acute care facility as this can increase a resident's risk of CDI. The NHSN therefore uses the date of last transfer from acute care facility to further subclassify LTCF-onset CDI LabID event to acute care transfer-LTCF onset (ACT-LO) CDI LabID event [2]. ACT-LO LabID events are LTCF-onset (LO) LabID events with date of specimen collection ≤4 weeks following date of last transfer from an acute care facility.

In addition to reporting CDI LabID events, facilities should also report monthly resident admissions, resident days, number of admissions on *C. difficile* treatment, and CDI treatment starts as these are used as denominators to calculate relevant CDI rates and metrics such as incidence rates, CDI treatment prevalence on admission, and CDI treatment ratio [2]. These rates and metrics can then be used to determine how *C. difficile* is manifest and transmitted in the LTCF setting and to compare rates with other LTCFs in the area and with national rates.

Alternatively, studies have used clinical definitions to determine the burden of CDI in LTCF [6, 7]. Clinical definitions require the presence of clinical symptoms consistent with CDI and either a positive laboratory diagnostic test result of a stool specimen or evidence of pseudomembranes demonstrated by endoscopy or histopathology [3]. Although clinical definitions probably provide a more accurate reflection of CDI burden in an LTCF, collection of data is much more labor intensive, and if data is collected retrospectively, lack of documentation of signs/symptoms in medical records may pose difficulty in case ascertainment.

Studies in acute care hospitals have shown good concordance between NHSN laboratory-based CDI definition and clinical CDI definition [8, 9]. Moreover, a study at a VA LTCF compared the incidence of CDI using NHSN surveillance definition with clinically defined CDI and found that the NHSN definition captured all the clinically defined CDI cases which had their onset and treatment in the LTCF itself [10]. However, the NHSN definition identified only 28% of the clinically defined CDI cases who were admitted to LTCF already diagnosed with and on therapy for CDI [10]. Calculating CDI treatment ratio (defined as number of CDI treatment starts/total number of CDI LabID events) will help capture the proportion of patients who were presumptively diagnosed with CDI and started on treatment without laboratory confirmation and those who did not receive CDI treatment despite a positive laboratory result likely due to inappropriately ordered test. The NHSN definition will also not capture residents with CDI transferred to acute care prior to being tested, but as noted in the earlier study, this will likely account for a small proportion of cases [10].

In conclusion, every LTCF facility should conduct CDI surveillance to determine how these organisms are manifest and transmitted in their facility. Analyzing the CDI rates detected by surveillance will help determine infection trends, detect outbreaks, and determine the impact of infection control and antibiotic stewardship interventions directed toward control of *C. difficile* [1, 2]. Use of standardized and widely available surveillance definitions such as those of NHSN will facilitate intra- and interfacility comparison of infection rates [2]. In addition, LTCFs should meet local, state, and national regulatory requirements for CDI reporting.

References

1. Smith PW, et al. SHEA/APIC guideline: infection prevention and control in the long-term care facility, July 2008. Infect Control Hosp Epidemiol. 2008;29(9):785–814.
2. Centers for Disease Control and Prevention. Laboratory-identified multidrug-resistant organism (MDRO) & Clostridium difficile infection (CDI) events for long-term care facilities (LTCFs).

3. McDonald LC, et al. Clinical practice guidelines for Clostridium difficile infection in adults and children: 2017 update by the Infectious Diseases Society of America (IDSA) and Society for Healthcare Epidemiology of America (SHEA). Clin Infect Dis. 2018;66(7):e1–e48.
4. Palms DL, et al. The National Healthcare Safety Network Long-term Care Facility Component early reporting experience: January 2013–December 2015. Am J Infect Control. 2018;46(6):637–42.
5. Stone ND. Post-Acute and Long Term Care: the changing national landscape. Presented at SHEA Spring Conference 2018.
6. Laffan AM, et al. Burden of Clostridium difficile-associated diarrhea in a long-term care facility. J Am Geriatr Soc. 2006;54(7):1068–73.
7. Gaynes R, et al. Outbreak of Clostridium difficile infection in a long-term care facility: association with gatifloxacin use. Clin Infect Dis. 2004;38(5):640–5.
8. Gase KA, et al. Comparison of 2 Clostridium difficile surveillance methods: National Healthcare Safety Network's laboratory-identified event reporting module versus clinical infection surveillance. Infect Control Hosp Epidemiol. 2013;34(3):284–90.
9. Kelly SG, et al. Inappropriate Clostridium difficile testing and consequent overtreatment and inaccurate publicly reported metrics. Infect Control Hosp Epidemiol. 2016;37(12):1395–400.
10. Han A, Jump RL. Discrepancies between surveillance definition and the clinical incidence of Clostridium difficile infection in a Veterans Affairs long-term care facility. Infect Control Hosp Epidemiol. 2014;35(11):1435–6.

Rishitha Bollam, Nisa Desai,
and Laurie Archbald-Pannone

Introduction

Clostridium difficile (*C. difficile*) infection (CDI) is the most common nosocomial infection and disproportionally affects our
elderly patients, with 80% of *C. difficile* infections occurring in
patients 65 years of age and older [1]. As described in other chapters of this book, patients with CDI can have multiple loose or
watery stools in 1 day causing extreme dehydration, electrolyte
disarray, sepsis, toxic megacolon, and even death. With the
increasing prevalence and severity of CDI over the past decade,

R. Bollam · N. Desai
University of Virginia, School of Medicine, Department of Internal
Medicine, Charlottesville, VA, USA

L. Archbald-Pannone (✉)
University of Virginia, School of Medicine, Department of Internal
Medicine, Division of General, Geriatric, Palliative & Hospital
Medicine, Charlottesville, VA, USA

University of Virginia, School of Medicine, Department of Internal
Medicine, Division of General, Geriatric, Palliative & Hospital Medicine
and Division of Infectious Diseases and International Health,
Charlottesville, VA, USA
e-mail: LA2E@hscmail.mcc.virginia.edu

© Springer Nature Switzerland AG 2020   45
T. Chopra (ed.), *Clostridium Difficile Infection in Long-Term Care
Facilities*, https://doi.org/10.1007/978-3-030-29772-5_5

clinicians are understandably concerned when suspecting CDI in one of their patients and keen to test to see if *C. difficile* is present in the stool. However, the presence of *C. difficile* in the stool is not sufficient to diagnose CDI, and the diagnostic tests currently commercially available for testing are complex. In 1935, Dr. Ivan Hall and Elizabeth O'Toole first identified and named *Clostridium difficile* (originally *Bacillus difficilis*) because the organism was difficult to isolate and grow in culture [2, 3]. CDI is a toxin-mediated infection and, therefore, diagnostic assays often focus on the presence of toxin as a necessary component to develop infection, as opposed to colonization with non-toxigenic *C. difficile* strain.

Clinical Manifestations of CDI

Patients with CDI must have loose and unformed stools. However, patients can also be asymptomatic carriers of *C. difficile*, and therefore, the clinical scenario in which a clinician decides to test for CDI is paramount to appropriate diagnosis. While CDI is common in the elderly and LTCF patients and the most common bacterial cause of acute diarrhea in this population, so too is asymptomatic carriage either upon facility admission or acquired during their stay [8].

Recent clinical guidelines for CDI cite that patients with suspicion of CDI must first have ≥3 unexplained and new-onset unformed stools in 24 hours [4]. There are many important pieces of this guideline statement to highlight here. First, patients much have diarrhea to be considered for CDI testing. Diarrhea is defined as an unformed stool that occurs at least three times within 1 day. Patients who are having formed stool should not be considered as having CDI, and therefore, clinical laboratories will refuse to test a formed stool specimen for *C. difficile*. A second notable part of the guidelines is that the unformed stool must be new and unexplained to be appropriate to consider for CDI testing. Therefore, a patient with a history of chronic diarrhea with no change from baseline is not appropriate for testing for CDI. As specifically detailed in the guideline, "If a patient has diarrheal symptoms not clearly attributable to underlying conditions (inflammatory bowel disease (IBD) and therapies such as enteral tube feeding, intensive cancer chemotherapy, or laxatives), then testing to determine if diarrhea is due to *C. difficile* is indicated. Alternatively, testing may be indicated if symptoms persist after stopping therapies to which diarrhea may be otherwise attributed (e.g., laxatives)" [4]. Therefore, all medical conditions, medications, and baseline stool history must be reviewed prior to consideration of *C. difficile* testing. Notably, patients with IBD and on enteral feeds are at increased risk for CDI, and thus, true infection should be suspected when these subgroups of patients have new or worsening diarrhea.

As described in previous chapters, it is critical to determine whether a patient has recently been exposed to antibiotics, as antibiotic disruption of microbiome remains the top risk factor for developing CDI. However, no recent history of antibiotic exposure has precluded the possibility of CDI in a patient with appropriate symptoms and other relevant risk factors for infection (e.g., age, recent hospitalization or stay in LTCF). Severe signs and symptoms of colitis could also aid in the diagnosis and often include lower quadrant pain, distension, and fevers. Typical laboratory evaluation reveals WBC > 15,000 and elevated serum creatinine >1.5 for severe disease. Fulminant disease is often characterized by hypotension, ileus, and megacolon. Lastly, CDI cause recurrent infections in which symptoms recur from days to months after completing appropriate CDI treatment.

Laboratory Testing

C. difficile is not typically cultured in the clinical laboratory, like other bacterium, due to the difficulty of culturing – hence the name *difficile*! [2, 3]. Instead, there are generally multiple types of diagnostic tests available to detect the *C. difficile*. Specifically, there are currently two reference standard assays commercially available for *C. difficile* testing; however, the utility for these testing is limited as they require a very high level of technical expertise. Cell cytotoxicity assay (CCTA) measures the presence of free *C. difficile* toxin (A or B) in the stool by detecting abolishment of cytopathic effect in cell culture by anti-toxin. This test has been shown to have a sensi tivity of 67–90% and is not often used due to the technical expertise required to properly conduct the assay. Cytotoxigenic culture (CC) requires culturing the bacterium from stool; if present, then it determines if the *C. difficile* strain present produces cytotoxins. This is considered the "gold standard" for testing in laboratory; however, it has limited utility in the clinical setting as isolating the bacterium is difficult and the turn-around time is not compatible with clinical need. Stool cultures alone – without toxin confirmation – has a low specificity due to prevalent asymptomatic carriage, especially in LTCFs [6, 8].

Enzyme immunoassay (EIA) testing has been commercially available for decades. These assays are rapid and do not require extensive technical expertise. These assays look for the presence of *gdh* or *tcd A/tcd B* – the genes that encode for glutamate dehydrogenase (GDH, *gdh*) [6]. GDH is a universal protein that is found in all strains of *C. difficile*. While this test is sensitive and useful to detect *C. difficile*, it is not able to differentiate between the toxigenic and non-toxigenic strains of *C. difficile*. GDH assays have a low specificity of 75–92% and a high sensitivity of 94.5% for true infection, necessitating it be used in combination with other assays [6].

There are numerous commercial tests available for CDI that look for the presence of one or both of the cytotoxins produced by *C. difficile* toxin B gene (*tcdB*) or toxin proteins. While EIA for *C. difficile* toxins A and B has a sensitivity of 69–99%, the test does have a very high specificity of 94–100% [6]. NAAT assay uses polymerase chain reaction (PCR) to identify the gene that encodes of toxin B (*tcdB*). Research has shown that clinically relevant CDI is caused by strains that produce either toxins A and B or toxin B alone [1]. However, while NAAT can determine the presence of toxin producing strain, it is not able to determine if there is active toxin production. Therefore, while this assay has a high specificity of 94–100% [6], it is unable to distinguish CDI from asymptomatic carriage. This limitation highlights the need to test stool only in appropriate clinical settings and scenarios.

Due to the diagnostic limitations of each individual testing modality, current *C. difficile* diagnostic guideline recommends using a multistep, algorithmic approach to *C. difficile* diagnosis [4]. Based on current guideline, the first step in CDI diagnosis is that clinicians and laboratory personnel should first agree on the appropriate patients and stool samples on which to do *C. difficile* testing – patients not on laxatives who have ≥3 new and unexplained unformed stools within 24 hours of testing [4]. If this agreement can be reached, then the recommended algorithm is NAAT alone (PCR for toxin) or stool toxin test (EIA) that has highest sensitivity reported [4], instead of toxin test alone. However, if clinicians and laboratory personnel do not have institutional agreement on diagnostic criteria, the guidelines instead recommend stool toxin assay as part of a multistep algorithm that can include GDH plus toxin if NAAT is positive or NAAT plus toxin assay, instead of just NAAT alone [4]. With proper diagnostic algorithm, repeat testing within 7 days of initial sample is not indicated [4].

To simplify these recommendations, optimal diagnostic testing for CDI is to use combined assay for GDH plus toxin with or without NAAT or use NAAT plus toxin assay. NAAT alone is not recommended without institutional criteria for stool specimen submission based on clinical criteria.

Consequences of False-Positive/-Negative Testing

It is necessary to choose the proper laboratory testing due to the consequences of false-positive or false-negative results.

False-positive testing – a patient tests negative for CDI but the laboratory tests are positive – will likely lead to a patient having increased and unnecessary CDI treatments with antibiotic that will further increase the patient's risk of ultimately developing CDI as well as developing antimicrobial resistance.

False-negative testing – a true case of CDI where the laboratory tests are negative – may lead to inappropriate discontinuation of CDI treatment and increased risk of poor outcome from infection, especially in a vulnerable elderly population.

Surveillance

Diagnostic surveillance for CDI in patients without diarrhea in LTCFs should not be done.

Clinicians and clinical staff must remain vigilant to determine if our patients develop diarrhea. CDI should be considered in our high-risk, LTCF, and elderly patients with appropriate clinical exposure who develop new diarrhea (defined as ≥3 unformed new and unexplained stools within 24 hours of testing). For these patients, prompt clinical and laboratory evaluation with appropriate testing should be performed.

Laboratory testing to determine resolution of infection should not be done. Resolution of CDI is determined based on clinical factors alone. Therefore, if a patient is treated for CDI and their diarrhea resolves, then there is no indication to test again for *C. difficile* to prove the patient is cured [4].

Patients with asymptomatic carriage do not need any further diagnostic testing as long as they remain asymptomatic [9].

Impact of *C. difficile* Testing on the Elderly and Long-Term Care Patient Populations

The elderly, especially in long-term care facilities (LTCFs), are at higher risk of developing infection as increasing age often leads to alterations of the gastrointestinal tract, changes in cellular and humoral immunity, and impaired immunoglobulin production. This allows for more frequent invasion of pathogens causing severe disease. While the majority of true *C. difficile* infections occur in adults 65 and older, a high proportion of LCTF patients are already colonized at the time of admission to the facility [8]. Thus, it becomes even more important to distinguish asymptomatic carriage from clinically significant disease in order to avoid unnecessary administration of antibiotics and breeding of resistance.

The diagnosis of CDI becomes more complicated in the elderly population, as they often do not mount as robust of an immune response to infection and thus do not have the typical systemic signs and symptoms of infection as aforementioned. It has been shown that fever is absent in 20–30% of the elderly as there is impaired thermoregulation with increasing age [5]. Interestingly, a non-specific decline in functional status noted by increasing confusion, falls, or anorexia is often a good surrogate marker for infection [7]. There is no doubt that having watery bowel movements is an important diagnostic component for CDI and is universal among all ages. Even in the absence of systemic signs and symptoms of infection, there should be a lower threshold to test for CDI in the elderly population, especially if they have a sudden decline in functional status.

References

1. Asempa TE, Nicolau DP. *Clostridium difficile* infection in the elderly: an update on management. Clin Interv Aging. 2017;12:1799.
2. EID Authors. Etymologia: *Clostridium difficile*. Emerg Infect Dis. 2010;16(4):674.
3. Hall IV, O'toole E. Intestinal Flora in new-born infants with description of a new pathogenic anaerobe, *Bacillus difficilis*. Am J Dis Child. 1935;49(2):390–402.
4. Mcdonald LC, Gerding DN, Johnson S, Bakken JS, Carroll KC, Coffin SE, Dubberke ER, Garey KW, Gould CV, Kelly C, Loo V. Clinical practice guidelines for *Clostridium difficile* infection in adults and children: 2017 update by the Infectious Diseases Society of America (IDSA) and Society for Healthcare Epidemiology of America (SHEA). Clin Infect Dis. 2018;66(7):e1–48.
5. Norman DC. Fever in the elderly. Clin Infect Dis. 2000;31(1):148–51.
6. Planche T, Wilcox MH. Diagnostic pitfalls in *Clostridium difficile* infection. Infect Dis Clin. 2015;29(1):63–82.
7. Rao K, Micic D, Chenoweth E, Deng L, Galecki AT, Ring C, Young VB, Aronoff DM, Malani PN. Poor functional status as a risk factor for severe *Clostridium difficile* infection in hospitalized older adults. J Am Geriatr Soc. 2013;61(10):1738–42.
8. Simor AE, Bradley SF, Strausbaugh LJ, Crossley K, Nicolle LE, SHEA Long-Term–Care Committee. *Clostridium difficile* in long-term–care facilities for the elderly. Infect Control Hosp Epidemiol. 2002;23(11):696–703.
9. Stone ND, Ashraf MS, Calder J, Crnich CJ, Crossley K, Drinka PJ, Gould CV, Juthani-Mehta M, Lautenbach E, Loeb M, MacCannell T. Surveillance definitions of infections in long-term care facilities: revisiting the McGeer criteria. Infect Control Hosp Epidemiol. 2012;33(10):965–77.

Control of *Clostridium* (*Clostridioides*) *difficile* Infection in Long-Term Care Facilities/Nursing Homes

6

Amar Krishna and Teena Chopra

In a healthcare setting, *Clostridium* (*Clostridioides*) *difficile* transmission most likely occurs as a result of person to person spread through the fecal-oral route or due to direct exposure to contaminated environment. The hands of healthcare personnel can become transiently contaminated with *C. difficile* spores and probably act as the main means by which the organism is spread in a healthcare setting [1]. Healthcare personnel can acquire the organism from patients with either active CDI or those who are asymptomatically colonized with *C. difficile* [2]. Patients with active *Clostridium difficile* infection (CDI) have large number of *C. difficile* spores in their stools, and healthcare personnel caring for these patients can unwittingly acquire the organism on their hands [3, 4]. As a result, most infection control interventions are directed against patients with active CDI. Although studies have shown that asymptomatically colonized patients with *C. difficile* contribute to CDI transmission, there is insufficient evidence to recommend screening for asymptomatic carriage and placing these patients in isolation in order to decrease CDI rates [2, 5]. Patients with recent CDI

A. Krishna (✉) · T. Chopra
Detroit Medical Center/Wayne State University, Detroit, MI, USA
e-mail: akrishn@med.wayne.edu

© Springer Nature Switzerland AG 2020
T. Chopra (ed.), *Clostridium Difficile Infection in Long-Term Care Facilities*, https://doi.org/10.1007/978-3-030-29772-5_6

might continue to shed large amount of *C. difficile* spores even after resolution of their diarrhea, indicating a population of asymptomatic carriers who are more likely to transmit the organism [6].

In a CDI endemic setting, acquisition through the contaminated environment likely accounts for only a small proportion of CDI cases [2]. Those that are particularly at risk are those admitted to rooms previously occupied by a CDI patient [3]. Even admission to a room where the previous patient was administered antibiotics but did not have CDI is a risk factor for symptomatic CDI [7]. In addition, various fomites have been implicated in *C. difficile* transmission and CDI outbreaks such as blood pressure cuffs, oral and rectal electronic thermometers, and contaminated commodes and bedpans [3, 8–10].

Infection control interventions are one of the cornerstones for prevention and control of *C. difficile* in a healthcare setting. These interventions have also been successfully used to control outbreaks of CDI in various healthcare settings [11–13]. Frequently, a bundle of infection control interventions such as hand hygiene, isolation measures, and environmental disinfection have been used, making it difficult to determine which interventions were most effective to control *C. difficile*. Most of these studies related to efficacy of infection control interventions have been performed in acute care hospitals [5]. Until more data specific to long-term care facilities (LTCFs) become available, these studies should serve as the basis for management of CDI in LTCFs [14].

Control of CDI in LTCFs provides unique set of challenges which are not encountered in acute care hospitals. LTCFs might be limited in personnel, expertise, and resources to implement antimicrobial stewardship and various infection control measures to control *C. difficile*. LTCFs might not have a private room available to isolate a patient who develops CDI. A survey in six LTCFs showed that only three LTCFs placed CDI residents in private rooms [15]. LTCFs also might have common toilets, bathrooms, rehabilitation, and dining and recreation areas which might prove a hindrance in implementing CDI specific infection control measures [16]. Even if resources are available, prolonged length of stay of LTCF residents and the need to provide home-like environment will limit implementation of some of the infection control measures [14, 16]. Many of the LTCF residents have dementia or other comorbid conditions which will limit their ability to adhere to basic standards of hygiene and contribute to organism spread. In addition, most LTCFs depend on off-site laboratories which might result in significant delays in CDI diagnosis.

LTCF staff also may have less collective knowledge and training regarding management of CDI. A 2005 survey in 248 Iowa LTCFs showed that 52% of LTCFs required both a negative *C. difficile* test and absence of diarrhea before discontinuing contact precautions [17]. Moreover, 77% of LTCFs tested for *C. difficile* only in the presence of complicated and severe diarrhea, therefore underestimating the true burden of infection [17]. Knowledge might be further reduced due to high staff turnover in these facilities especially if the new incoming staff are not educated and trained at recruitment [18].

In order to overcome these challenges, infection control measures recommended for acute care hospitals should be modified to suit the LTCF setting. In addition, LTCFs should collaborate with regional acute care hospitals in order to obtain the required expertise to manage CDI and obtain information on a patient's CDI status at the time of care transitions. All LTCFs should also have evidence-based written infection control policies specifically addressing *C. difficile* which should be updated at least on an annual basis.

The following discussion focuses on recommended control measures for *C. difficile* and the potential strategies to adapt them in an LTCF setting. The strength of recommendation and quality of evidence for various infection control measures are noted in Table 6.1.

Avoid Delays in CDI Diagnosis

LTCFs should empower physician assistants, nurse practitioners, and nurses to order *C. difficile* test if clinical criteria are met [19]. LTCFs should ensure timely collection and transport of stool samples to the laboratory. LTCFs frequently rely on off-site laborato

Table 6.1 Rating the quality of evidence and strength of recommendation using GRADE (Grading of Recommendation, Assessment, Development and Evaluation) methodology [40] for various CDI infection control measures

Patient isolation	Strong recommendation, moderate quality of evidence
Glove use	Strong recommendation, high quality of evidence
Gown use	Strong recommendation, moderate quality of evidence
Hand hygiene, endemic setting	Strong recommendation, moderate quality of evidence
Hand hygiene, outbreak/ hyperendemic setting	Weak recommendation, low quality of evidence
Patient bathing	Good practice recommendation
Environmental cleaning	Weak recommendation, low quality of evidence
Evaluating cleaning efficacy	Good practice recommendation
Disposable and dedicated equipment	Strong recommendation, moderate quality of evidence

ries for *C. difficile* testing which might result in significant delays in CDI diagnosis causing delay in starting therapy and implementation of infection control measures [16]. This could contribute to *C. difficile* transmission in the LTCF. LTCFs should therefore create an alert system with off-site laboratories to notify positive *C. difficile* results or inquire laboratories on a daily basis [16]. If results cannot be obtained on the same day, then LTCFs should place patients with suspected CDI on isolation while the results of *C. difficile* testing are awaited [5]. Consideration should also be given to starting empiric treatment for *C. difficile* if significant delays in laboratory confirmation are anticipated [5].

Lower Threshold to Test for *C. difficile*

A significant percentage of CDI cases go undiagnosed [20]. LTCFs should therefore have a low threshold to test for *C. difficile*. Any resident with unexplained diarrhea especially during or immediately after completing a course of antibiotic therapy should be suspected of having CDI [5, 19]. In a study involving acute care hospitals, LTCFs and outpatient clinics showed that facilities which were testing more frequently had lower prevalence of CDI compared to those facilities that infrequently tested for *C. difficile* [21]. Increased *C. difficile* testing likely leads to increased case detection and prompts institution of prevention measures and treatment limiting organism spread which eventually lead to decrease in CDI prevalence [21].

Education

Healthcare personnel in LTCFs should be educated about transmission, clinical features, diagnosis, management, and prevention of CDI [22]. LTCF personnel should be educated at least annually. If high staff turnover is anticipated, then more frequent education is needed to update new recruits [16].

Private Rooms or Cohorting for CDI Patients

Private rooms for CDI patients likely facilitate better infection control practices and result in decreased transmission to other residents [5]. Patients housed in double rooms have higher rates of CDI compared to those in single rooms, and roommates of CDI patients are more likely to acquire the organism [3]. Patients with CDI should be cared for in a private room with a dedicated toilet. If private rooms are limited, then CDI patients with fecal incontinence should be prioritized to placement in these rooms [5]. If private rooms are not available as the case may be in LTCFs, then CDI patients can be cohorted in the same room with dedicated commodes provided to each resident. When cohorting is done, colonization with other multidrug-resistant pathogens (methicillin-resistant *Staphylococcus aureus*, vancomycin-resistant *Enterococcus*) needs to be noted, and patients colonized with similar pathogens should be cohorted together [5]. If isolation in private rooms and cohorting cannot be done, then contact precautions can be maintained in multi-bed rooms with education of staff [16].

Contact Precautions (Use of Gloves and Gown)

During CDI patient care, hands of healthcare personnel are frequently contaminated by *C. difficile* spores which can later be transmitted to other patients in their care [1, 3]. Hand hygiene and glove use during patient contact will decrease the concentration of spores in the hands of healthcare personnel, thus reducing risk of CDI transmission. One study showed use of vinyl gloves in handling body substances reduced CDI incidence in the intervention wards but not in control wards where glove use was not implemented [23]. Another study in an LTCF showed that it was unlikely to find *C. difficile* in hands of healthcare personnel who regularly washed hands and used gloves [24]. Because of its proven efficacy, gloves should be used for caring all CDI patients, when entering their rooms or handling their body substances.

Healthcare workers' uniforms can be contaminated by *C. difficile* spores; however, it is unknown if such contamination contributes to the spread of CDI [25]. Efficacy of disposable gowns in reducing CDI transmission is unclear since this intervention has been implemented together with other infection control measures, making it difficult to assess its effectiveness. Despite the uncertain benefits, experts recommend using disposable gowns while caring for patients with CDI [5]. Gloves and gowns should be made readily available near CDI patient rooms and should include signage that illustrates their proper use [16].

As per the new guidelines, isolation measures (private rooms/cohorting and contact precautions) should be continued for at least 48 hours after diarrhea resolves [5]. The guidelines also recommend extending isolation precautions until discharge if CDI rates remain high despite adherence to standard infection control measures [5]. This might not be feasible in LTCFs due to prolonged length of stay of residents and need to provide home-like environment [16]. Therefore, extending isolation in LTCF residents should be made on an individual basis and should be considered if these residents are believed to be a significant source of *C. difficile* transmission.

Hand Hygiene

Hand hygiene is one of the most important measures to prevent transmission of *C. difficile* and other healthcare-associated infections. Hand hygiene with soap and water will aid in physically removing the *C. difficile* spores from the hands of healthcare personnel. Studies have shown that it is less likely to find *C. difficile* in hands of healthcare workers who perform regular hand washing [24]. Studies have also noted low rate of handwashing by healthcare personnel [26]. Alcohol-based hand rubs are increasingly being used to improve compliance with hand hygiene in healthcare facilities. Although there is a theoretical concern that use of alcohol-based products for hand hygiene might increase CDI rates (since alcohol is not sporicidal and will not eliminate *C. difficile* spores from the hands but simply displace them), studies have not shown use of such products will increase CDI incidence [27, 28].

Therefore, during CDI endemic settings, the guidelines recommend the use of either soap and water or alcohol-based hand hygiene product before and after caring for a CDI patient or after contact with the patient's environment [5]. During outbreak or hyperendemic settings, handwashing with soap and water is preferred to alcohol-based products as alcohol might not reliably remove/inhibit *C. difficile* spores [5]. Handwashing with soap and water is also preferred when hands are visibly soiled and when there is contact with feces or with area where fecal contamination is likely [5]. LTCFs should provide staff with accessible handwashing facilities and make alcohol-based hand hygiene products readily available. Although it can be time consuming and require resources, LTCFs should monitor compliance with hand hygiene and contact precautions and share results with staff (only a few assessments can be done on an intermittent basis) [16].

Resident Handwashing and Bathing

The hands of CDI patients can become contaminated with *C. difficile* [29]. These patients can in turn transmit spores to surfaces or could ingest spores. The latter could lead to CDI recurrence.

Other body surfaces of CDI patients could also become contaminated with *C. difficile* spores [6]. Compared to bed bathing, showering has been shown to reduce skin contamination with *C. difficile* [30]. Therefore, the guidelines encourage patients to wash hands with soap and water and shower to decrease the concentration of *C. difficile* spores on hands and other skin surfaces, respectively [5]. If LTCF residents with CDI can wash hands and shower, they should be encouraged to do so.

Environmental Disinfection

Patients who have CDI or colonized with *C. difficile* shed spores and contaminate the local environment [31]. *C. difficile* spores are more likely to be found in rooms of patients with CDI than in rooms of patients who are colonized with *C. difficile* or in rooms where patients neither have CDI nor are colonized [31]. Spores can be found on bed rails, bed sheets, floors, toilets, commodes, bedpans, sinks, and many other sites in rooms of patients [4, 31, 32]. Studies also show that degree of environmental contamination correlates with degree of healthcare personnel hand contamination with *C. difficile* spores [4]. Therefore, the room of CDI patients should be cleaned and disinfected in order to reduce spore burden and prevent transmission. However, *C. difficile* spores are resistant to commonly used disinfectants; only sporicidal agents (such as chlorine-based compounds) have been shown to reduce surface contamination with *C. difficile* [33]. Despite the efficacy of sporicidal agents in reducing *C. difficile* spore burden, this does not necessarily result in reduced CDI incidence in an endemic setting, likely because the degree of environmental contamination is not high enough to cause transmission [34]. The reduction in CDI incidence with the use of sporicidal agents has been noted, however, in the setting of CDI outbreaks or hyperendemic CDI rates when combined with other interventions to prevent CDI [35, 36]. Therefore, the guidelines only recommend the use of sporicidal agents in these scenarios or when there is evidence of repeated cases of CDI from the same room indicating extensive environmental contamination with *C. difficile spores* [5].

In the LTCF setting, resources and personnel might not permit daily disinfection of CDI patient rooms with sporicidal agents. As these agents are also of unproven efficacy in an endemic setting, these should only be considered as supplemental interventions in an LTCF. Standard facility cleaning protocol should be followed in CDI patient rooms as well and adequacy of cleaning monitored.

Evaluate Cleaning Efficacy

Several methods such as fluorescent markers and adenosine tri-phosphate bioluminescence have been used to assess cleaning efficacy [37, 38]. These methods correlate well with microbiologic methods of cleaning efficacy and are most effective when feedback is given in real time [38, 39]. However, these methods might be expensive and time consuming if implemented in LTCFs. LTCFs could consider inexpensive methods such as use of fluorescent markers and/or evaluate cleaning efficacy on an intermittent basis in only a few randomly selected rooms [16]. Educating environmental staff about proper cleaning methods and providing them with adequate cleaning supplies are also crucial.

Use Disposable and Dedicated Equipment

Blood pressure cuffs and oral and rectal electronic thermometers have been implicated in CDI outbreaks [8, 9]. Incidence of CDI has been reduced with the use of disposable thermometers in place of reusable electronic thermometers [9, 10]. These results support the use of disposable equipment when possible. Nondisposable equipment such as blood pressure cuffs and stethoscopes should be dedicated to the patient's room [5]. If equipment is to be reused after use in a CDI patient, then it must be cleaned and disinfected preferably with a sporicidal agent that is equipment compatible [5]. The facility's policy should clearly mention the personnel (environmental services vs nurses/nurses' aides) responsible for cleaning and disinfection of equipment. LTCF residents with CDI who have rehabilitation needs should be encouraged to use rehabilitation equipment at the end of the day [16]. The equipment should then be thoroughly cleaned and disinfected before use by other residents the following day.

The implementation of the above-mentioned infection control measures in a specific LTCF would depend on the burden of CDI in that facility. Basic measures such as hand hygiene, glove use, environmental cleaning, and isolation/cohorting should be implemented in most LTCFs. Additional control measures can then be added if CDI rates fail to improve despite proper adherence with the measures that are already in place.

References

1. Bobulsky GS, et al. *Clostridium difficile* skin contamination in patients with *C. difficile*-associated disease. Clin Infect Dis. 2008;46(3):447–50.
2. Curry SR, et al. Use of multilocus variable number of tandem repeats analysis genotyping to determine the role of asymptomatic carriers in *Clostridium difficile* transmission. Clin Infect Dis. 2013;57(8): 1094–102.
3. McFarland LV, et al. Nosocomial acquisition of *Clostridium difficile* infection. N Engl J Med. 1989;320(4):204–10.
4. Samore MH, et al. Clinical and molecular epidemiology of sporadic and clustered cases of nosocomial *Clostridium difficile* diarrhea. Am J Med. 1996;100(1):32–40.
5. McDonald LC, et al. Clinical practice guidelines for *Clostridium difficile* infection in adults and children: 2017 update by the Infectious Diseases Society of America (IDSA) and Society for Healthcare Epidemiology of America (SHEA). Clin Infect Dis. 2018;66(7):e1–e48.
6. Sethi AK, et al. Persistence of skin contamination and environmental shedding of *Clostridium difficile* during and after treatment of C. difficile infection. Infect Control Hosp Epidemiol. 2010;31(1):21–7.
7. Freedberg DE, et al. Receipt of antibiotics in hospitalized patients and risk for *Clostridium difficile* infection in subsequent patients who occupy the same bed. JAMA Intern Med. 2016;176(12):1801–8.
8. Manian FA, Meyer L, Jenne J. *Clostridium difficile* contamination of blood pressure cuffs: a call for a closer look at gloving practices in the era of universal precautions. Infect Control Hosp Epidemiol. 1996;17(3):180–2.
9. Brooks SE, et al. Reduction in the incidence of *Clostridium difficile*-associated diarrhea in an acute care hospital and a skilled nursing facility following replacement of electronic thermometers with single-use disposables. Infect Control Hosp Epidemiol. 1992;13(2):98–103.

10. Jernigan JA, et al. A randomized crossover study of disposable thermometers for prevention of *Clostridium difficile* and other nosocomial infections. Infect Control Hosp Epidemiol. 1998;19(7):494–9.

11. Muto CA, et al. Control of an outbreak of infection with the hypervirulent *Clostridium difficile* BI strain in a university hospital using a comprehensive "bundle" approach. Clin Infect Dis. 2007;45(10):1266–73.

12. Weiss K, et al. Multipronged intervention strategy to control an outbreak of *Clostridium difficile* infection (CDI) and its impact on the rates of CDI from 2002 to 2007. Infect Control Hosp Epidemiol. 2009;30(2):156–62.

13. Cassir N, et al. A regional outbreak of *Clostridium difficile* PCR-ribotype 027 infections in southeastern France from a single long-term care facility. Infect Control Hosp Epidemiol. 2016;37(11):1337–41.

14. Simor AE, et al. *Clostridium difficile* in long-term-care facilities for the elderly. Infect Control Hosp Epidemiol. 2002;23(11):696–703.

15. Archbald-Pannone L. Survey of C. difficile-specific infection control policies in local long-term care facilities. Int J Clin Med. 2014;5(7):414–9.

16. Jump RL, Donskey CJ. *Clostridium difficile* in the long-term care facility: prevention and management. Curr Geriatr Rep. 2015;4(1):60–9.

17. Quinn LK, Chen Y, Herwaldt LA. Infection control policies and practices for Iowa long-term care facility residents with *Clostridium difficile* infection. Infect Control Hosp Epidemiol. 2007;28(11):1228–32.

18. AHCA. American Health Care Association 2012 staffing report. http://www.ahcancal.org/research_data/staffing/Documents/2012_Staffing_Report.pdf. Accessed 14 Apr 2019.

19. Chopra T, Goldstein EJ. *Clostridium difficile* infection in long-term care facilities: a call to action for antimicrobial stewardship. Clin Infect Dis. 2015;60(Suppl 2):S72–6.

20. Davies KA, et al. Underdiagnosis of *Clostridium difficile* across Europe: the European, multicentre, prospective, biannual, point-prevalence study of *Clostridium difficile* infection in hospitalised patients with diarrhoea (EUCLID). Lancet Infect Dis. 2014;14(12):1208–19.

21. Krishna A, et al. Prevalence of *Clostridium difficile* infection in acute care hospitals, long-term care facilities, and outpatient clinics: is *Clostridium difficile* infection underdiagnosed in long-term care facility patients? Am J Infect Control. 2017;45(10):1157–9.

22. Simor AE. Diagnosis, management, and prevention of *Clostridium difficile* infection in long-term care facilities: a review. J Am Geriatr Soc. 2010;58(8):1556–64.

23. Johnson S, et al. Prospective, controlled study of vinyl glove use to interrupt *Clostridium difficile* nosocomial transmission. Am J Med. 1990;88(2):137–40.

24. Larson E, et al. Lack of care giver hand contamination with endemic bacterial pathogens in a nursing home. Am J Infect Control. 1992;20(1):11–5.

25. Perry C, Marshall R, Jones E. Bacterial contamination of uniforms. J Hosp Infect. 2001;48(3):238–41.

26. Pittet D, Mourouga P, Perneger TV. Compliance with handwashing in a teaching hospital. Infection Control Program. Ann Intern Med. 1999;130(2):126–30.

27. Oughton MT, et al. Hand hygiene with soap and water is superior to alcohol rub and antiseptic wipes for removal of *Clostridium difficile*. Infect Control Hosp Epidemiol. 2009;30(10):939–44.

28. Gordin FM, et al. Reduction in nosocomial transmission of drug-resistant bacteria after introduction of an alcohol-based handrub. Infect Control Hosp Epidemiol. 2005;26(7):650–3.

29. Kundrapu S, et al. More cleaning, less screening: evaluation of the time required for monitoring versus performing environmental cleaning. Infect Control Hosp Epidemiol. 2014;35(2):202–4.

30. Jury LA, et al. Effectiveness of routine patient bathing to decrease the burden of spores on the skin of patients with *Clostridium difficile* infection. Infect Control Hosp Epidemiol. 2011;32(2):181–4.

31. Kim KH, et al. Isolation of *Clostridium difficile* from the environment and contacts of patients with antibiotic-associated colitis. J Infect Dis. 1981;143(1):42–50.

32. Fawley WN, Wilcox MH. Molecular epidemiology of endemic *Clostridium difficile* infection. Epidemiol Infect. 2001;126(3):343–50.

33. Fawley WN, et al. Efficacy of hospital cleaning agents and germicides against epidemic *Clostridium difficile* strains. Infect Control Hosp Epidemiol. 2007;28(8):920–5.

34. Mayfield JL, et al. Environmental control to reduce transmission of *Clostridium difficile*. Clin Infect Dis. 2000;31(4):995–1000.

35. Kaatz GW, et al. Acquisition of *Clostridium difficile* from the hospital environment. Am J Epidemiol. 1988;127(6):1289–94.

36. McMullen KM, et al. Use of hypochlorite solution to decrease rates of *Clostridium difficile*-associated diarrhea. Infect Control Hosp Epidemiol. 2007;28(2):205–7.

37. Sitzlar B, et al. An environmental disinfection odyssey: evaluation of sequential interventions to improve disinfection of *Clostridium difficile* isolation rooms. Infect Control Hosp Epidemiol. 2013;34(5):459–65.

38. Boyce JM, et al. Monitoring the effectiveness of hospital cleaning practices by use of an adenosine triphosphate bioluminescence assay. Infect Control Hosp Epidemiol. 2009;30(7):678–84.

39. Munoz-Price LS, et al. Decreasing operating room environmental pathogen contamination through improved cleaning practice. Infect Control Hosp Epidemiol. 2012;33(9):897–904.

40. US GRADE Network. Approach and implications to rating the quality of evidence and strength of recommendations using the GRADE methodology, 2015. Available at: http://www.gradeworkinggroup.org/.

Antibiotic Stewardship Related to CDI in Long-Term Care Facilities

7

Bhagyashri D. Navalkele

Introduction

Clostridioides difficile (previous name *Clostridium difficile*) is a major burden to the healthcare system with an unaccountable contribution from long-term care facilities (LTCF) [1]. To reduce this burden, every year Joint Commission standards have recognized prevention of *Clostridioides difficile infection* (CDI) as one of the National Patient Safety Goals. Generally, most of the focus remains on prevention measures such as strict isolation, hand hygiene with soap and water, and environmental disinfection to reduce CDI transmission. These measures are restricted in application to a group of patients with suspected or confirmed CDI. The key strategy to prevent *C. difficile* colonization, even prior to the manifestation of infection, is reducing inappropriate antibiotic use.

B. D. Navalkele (✉)
University of Mississippi Medical Center, Jackson, MS, USA

© Springer Nature Switzerland AG 2020   65
T. Chopra (ed.), *Clostridium Difficile Infection in Long-Term Care Facilities*, https://doi.org/10.1007/978-3-030-29772-5_7

Need for Antimicrobial Stewardship in Long-Term Care Facilities

Exposure to antibiotics in previous 3 months, multiple courses of antibiotic therapy, and length of antibiotic treatment alter the gut flora and are associated with high risk for *C. difficile* colonization [2]. Even a single dose of high-risk antimicrobials such as clindamycin, fluoroquinolones, and cephalosporins increases risk for CDI.

Commonly, LTCF residents have complex medical conditions lowering their threshold to antibiotic exposure. Residents receive at least one course of antibiotic every year [3]. Old age and rise in antibiotic utilization have resulted in high *C. difficile* acquisition rates (8–33%) at LTCFs [3]. Current estimated CDI incidence rate in LTCF is 2.3 cases/10,000 resident days [4].

To combat antibiotic-resistant bacteria and infections, the White House released a national action plan to achieve a goal of 50% reduction in incidence of CDI by 2020. Effectively, the Centers for Medicare and Medicaid Services (CMS) proposed regulatory rule to implement antimicrobial stewardship programs in all hospital settings including LTCF [2].

Since the regulatory advent, acute care hospital data is the strongest evidence on the effectiveness of stewardship programs. A multidisciplinary stewardship program in an acute care hospital setting reported a significant decrease in CDI rates ($p = 0.002$) sustained over a 7-year period by limiting utilization of third-generation cephalosporins [5]. A systematic review and meta-analysis of 16 studies restricting cephalosporin and fluoroquinolone use showed protective benefit with a 52% risk reduction in CDI cases [6]. Following a CDI outbreak at a VA facility, Climo et al. performed a prospective cohort study observing the effect of restriction of clindamycin use on CDI rates. The study reported sustained reduction in CDI cases (11.5 cases/month compared with 3.33 cases/month; $p < 0.001$) and cost savings (an estimated $47,782 by preventing 237 CDI cases) over a 3-year time period [7]. Successful reduction in CDI rates post-emergence of robust antibiotic stewardship programs "(ASPs)" in an acute care setting supplements as a strong need for similar action in LTCFs.

ABCs of Antimicrobial Stewardship Program

Antimicrobial or antibiotic stewardship (ASP) entitles efficient antibiotic utilization for an appropriate indication with the right antibiotic, at right dose and route of administration, and for a right duration of time. The primary objective of ASP is to establish a multidisciplinary team to promote education and awareness on increasing antimicrobial resistance, implement policies, and monitor the appropriate use of antibiotics. The scope of ASP is vast, extending beyond prevention of CDI to the reduction in incidence of other multidrug-resistant organisms (MDROs) and antibiotic-associated adverse events, reducing healthcare expenditures through antibiotic cost savings, and overall improving patient care, safety, and quality of life.

As LTCF system differs from acute care hospitals, multidisciplinary expert panels from the Society for Healthcare Epidemiology of America (SHEA), Association for Professionals in Infection Control (APIC), and Infectious Diseases Society of America (IDSA) recommend infection preventionists in LTCFs to step up and incorporate antimicrobial stewardship activities in the infection control programs (Category IB) [2]. The guidance tool published by the Centers for Disease Control and Prevention (CDC) recognized as a standard to establish ASP at any acute care and long-term care facility [8]. Table 7.1 highlights core elements in stewardship with specific recommendations directed to LTCFs on gradual implementation of strategies over time for stability and sustainment of stewardship program.

Barriers in Long-Term Care Facilities

Despite comprehensive guidance, hardly 25–60% of LTCFs have formal ASPs [9]. Majority of these programs lack written policies, financial and leadership support, as well as dedicated staffing. Infection prevention personnel commonly leads stewardship efforts without adequate support. The facility-based ASPs perform limited basic activities such as monitoring antibiotic use,

Table 7.1 Core elements of antimicrobial stewardship program

Core elements	Stakeholders	Goals and objectives
Commitment Key element for success of program	Administrative leadership Clinical leadership: medical director, director of nursing services, director of staff development Infectious disease specialist Infection prevention and healthcare epidemiology staff Pharmacist Microbiology Information technology	Goal: To establish and sustain ASP Objectives: –Provide formal written statement of support to improve and monitor antibiotic use –Provide financial support for stewardship activities –Include stewardship duties as part of work requirement and annual performance review –Support for staff training and education –Support for stewardship activities with engagement of multidisciplinary group

Accountability	Physician leader, preferably infectious diseases trained	Goal: To lead and monitor stewardship program Objectives: –Establish stewardship committee/workgroup composing infection preventionist (must), nursing director, medical director, consulting pharmacist, administrator, physician champion, nurse champion, nurse aide champion, and resident and family council representative –Plan, develop, and implement stewardship policies, procedures, and protocol –Direct communication and feedback to providers and staff on adherence to antimicrobial prescribing per policy –Review and monitor outcomes of stewardship activities
Drug expertise	Pharmacy leader as co-champion	Goal: To co-lead, promote, monitor, and support stewardship activities Objectives: –Develop facility-specific antibiogram based on local susceptibility pattern –Participate in development of stewardship policies, procedures, and protocol –Review adherence to antibiotic prescribing policy –Provide recommendations to stewardship committee/workgroup based on outcomes and resistance data

(continued)

Table 7.1 (continued)

Core elements	Stakeholders	Goals and objectives
Action	Antimicrobial stewardship committee	Goal: To implement strategies to improve antibiotic use
		Objectives:
		–Perform baseline assessment on antibiotic prescribing practices for common infections, average duration of antibiotic treatment, and CDI rate.
		–Identify simple, measurable, and modifiable targets to review and monitor change in antibiotic use before and after ASP intervention.
		–Routine communication of implemented policies, procedures, and protocols with all providers and staff
		–Recommend LTCFs to implement at least one of the below measurable strategies during start of ASP:
		*Publish antibiotic prescription policy advising providers to include dose, duration, and indication for each recommended antibiotic
		*Publish facility specific guidelines on treatment of CDI based on severity. Include treatment of other common infections (urinary tract infection, pneumonia, skin and soft tissue infection, invasive infections) in guidelines
		*Provide guidance on ordering appropriate diagnostic studies based on clinical assessment (e.g., C. *difficile* PCR, toxin assay)
		*Provide access to standard published guidelines on recommended duration of antibiotic treatment
		*Implement antibiotic time-out/stop protocol to promote 48–72 hours reassessment of appropriate antibiotic use based on clinical and diagnostic evaluation
		*Implement prior authorization to reduce inappropriate antibiotic use
		*Optimize antibiotic use by providing prospective audit and feedback to providers
		*Empower pharmacy-led initiatives to automate optimal antibiotic dosing, route of administration, and evaluation of drug-drug interactions

Tracking and reporting	Antimicrobial stewardship committee	Goal: To periodically monitor, track, and report outcome measures within the committee and annual review with staff and providers Objectives: Track and monitor at least one of the below outcome measures, corresponding to implemented strategy, to analyze success of the ASP: –Antibiotic use: measure days of therapy/1000 resident days of care –Change in CDI rate: based on restriction of high risk antibiotics –Cost savings: antibiotic costs, healthcare costs –Adherence to facility specific treatment guidelines –Prevalence of antibiotic resistance
Education	Physician providers, prescribers, clinical staff Nursing staff Residents and family	Goal: To educate, raise awareness, and obtain support to improve antibiotic use and reduce CDI Objectives: –Educate physicians and nursing staff on cause–effect relationship of improper use of antibiotics, development of antibiotic resistance, and rise in CDI rates –Review published facility-specific guidelines and protocols with staff (in the form of didactic presentations, posters, flyers, reminders) on appropriate antibiotic use –Provide feedback on facility-wide antibiotic use and to individual providers on antibiotic utilization per policy –Provide education to residents and families during admission to facility (in the form of posters, flyers, and direct communication) on ASP in an effort to improve antibiotic use and reduce facility-onset infections particularly CDI

appropriateness, providing antibiogram, and tracking CDI rates. Thus, partial implementation of core elements has resulted in unstable and poorly sustained ASP in LTCFs. The major barriers for stewardship deficiencies in LTCFs include remote facilities with lack of on-site infectious diseases trained physician, lack of specialized pharmacist, and lack of diagnostic resources such as on-site microbiology lab [9]. Poor staff knowledge on stewardship, poor response by providers to inappropriate prescribing practices, less engaged physician and staff in stewardship initiatives, and antibiotic pressure by patient/family have attributed to failure of stewardship initiatives [10, 11]. Overall, limited resources, complex patient population, and different culture of practice in LTCFs prohibit successful implementation and sustainment of ASP.

Recommended Solutions and Resources to Overcome Barriers

Few studies have explored barriers in LTCFs to provide guidance on practical solutions and resources to facilitate ASP. The Society for Post-Acute and Long-Term Care Medicine developed an antibiotic stewardship policy template, specific for LTCFs [12]. The policy provides guidance on implementation of ASP to meet CMS requirements. Acknowledging the lack of physician availability, the policy promotes use of provider-friendly algorithms like revised McGeer criteria and Loeb minimum criteria to diagnose common infections per surveillance definitions and to determine need for initiation of antibiotic therapy. Additional simple guidance to promote appropriate antibiotic use in LTCF is provided by Zarowitz et al. using treatment algorithms tailored toward infections commonly encountered in older adults (urinary tract infections, upper respiratory tract infections, pneumonia, skin and soft tissue infections) [13].

Alternative recommended strategy to prevent CDI is gaining consultation from infectious diseases (ID) expert. A 160-bed VA based LTCF showed a 30% reduction in total antimicrobial use and a significant reduction in CDI rate ($p = 0.04$) post-implementation of ID consultation services [14]. Appointing an ID expert by individual LTCF or group of LTCFs can be an effective way to combat antimicrobial usage in resource-limited setting.

One of the important overlooked cause for continued high burden of CDI in healthcare facilities is the constant transfer of residents from LTCFs to acute care hospitals (ACH) and vice versa. Thus, strong ASPs in LTCFs will make a major impact in reducing overall CDI rates. A 212-bed LTCF in Massachusetts collaborated with local ACH to obtain stewardship support via telemedicine. The local ASP team led by infectious diseases expert conducted daily chart reviews, generated reports on antimicrobial use, and gave feedback to LTCF providers through emails. Three-year post-implementation results demonstrated a reduction in high-risk antimicrobial use and hospital-acquired CDI rates ($p = 0.02$) [15]. Another LTCF collaborated with the local hospital-based ASP to promote education to physicians, staff, pharmacist, and resident family members on appropriate antibiotic use. On a 12-month follow-up, the LTCF reported reduced fluoroquinolone use by 37% but with non-significant reduction in CDI incidence by 19% [16]. There is a strong need for such collaborations to mitigate staffing and financial issues promoting utility of infectious diseases and pharmacy consultations from local ACHs for stewardship activities. Ultimately, these collaborations reduce overall burden of infections and antibiotic resistance in community and thus increase sustainability of ASP in LTCF.

Impact of Stewardship in Long-Term Care Facilities on CDI Rates

Outcome studies published since the implementation of ASP in LTCFs have reported simultaneous reduction in CDI rates and improvement in antimicrobial use [17, 18]. Limited studies have specifically analyzed reduction in the CDI rates. A 50-bed LTCF in the southeast United States reported a 23% reduction in CDI rates sustained over a 1-year period. The facility had successful reduction in CDI by implementing a tiered approach including infection prevention and stewardship measures reducing general antibiotic use and restricting use of clindamycin and cephalosporins [19]. Bunch et al. reported institution of ASP in addition to ongoing infection prevention measures in a 55-bed LTCF. During the 6-year study period, there was a 33% reduction in antibiotic cost per patient day, and CDI SIR rate reduced from 1.25 to 0.25 (two-tailed p-value = 0.0009) [20]. Valiquette et al. reported significant decline in CDI cases ($p = 0.007$) with establishment of stewardship program reducing high-risk antimicrobial use (cephalosporins, ciprofloxacin, clindamycin, macrolides), post-failure of impact of infection prevention strategies [21]. Few studies have reported no significant impact of stewardship efforts on CDI outcomes. Two LTCFs reported 21–25% reduction in antimicrobial use secondary to stewardship interventions. However, both studies observed no change in CDI rates [22]. Inapt impact of stewardship on CDI outcomes has been attributed to inadequate infection prevention measures [23].

Summary

Compared to acute care hospital setting, establishing and maintaining ASP in LTCF remains a challenge. Leadership support, staff education, and routine review and feedback by engaged ASP leaders are the essential pillars for the success of stewardship program. Reduction in CDI, particularly, necessitates multidisciplinary, bundled approach and collaboration with infection prevention to produce an impact. There is a need for further research on effective ways to sustain stewardship program and improve outcome measures in the resource-limited LTCFs.

References

1. Dubberke ER, Olsen MA. Burden of Clostridium difficile on the healthcare system. Clin Infect Dis. 2012;55(Suppl 2):S88–92.
2. Smith PW, Bennett G, Bradley S, Drinka P, Lautenbach E, Marx J, et al. SHEA/APIC guideline: infection prevention and control in the long-term care facility, July 2008. Infect Control Hosp Epidemiol. 2008;29(9):785–814.

3. Chopra T, Goldstein EJ. Clostridium difficile infection in long-term care facilities: a call to action for antimicrobial stewardship. Clin Infect Dis. 2015;60(Suppl 2):S72–6.
4. Pawar D, Tsay R, Nelson DS, Elumalai MK, Lessa FC, Clifford McDonald L, et al. Burden of Clostridium difficile infection in long-term care facilities in Monroe County, New York. Infect Control Hosp Epidemiol. 2012;33(11):1107–12.
5. Carling P, Fung T, Killion A, Terrin N, Barza M. Favorable impact of a multidisciplinary antibiotic management program conducted during 7 years. Infect Control Hosp Epidemiol. 2003;24(9):699–706.
6. Feazel LM, Malhotra A, Perencevich EN, Kaboli P, Diekema DJ, Schweizer ML. Effect of antibiotic stewardship programmers on Clostridium difficile incidence: a systematic review and meta-analysis. J Antimicrob Chemother. 2014;69(7):1748–54.
7. Climo MW, Israel DS, Wong ES, Williams D, Coudron P, Markowitz SM. Hospital-wide restriction of clindamycin: effect on the incidence of Clostridium difficile-associated diarrhea and cost. Ann Intern Med. 1998;128(12 Pt 1):989–95.
8. Centers for Disease Control and Prevention. Core elements of hospital antibiotic stewardship programs. Atlanta: US Department of Health and Human Services, CDC; 2014. Accessed 30 Sept 2014.
9. Morrill HJ, Caffrey AR, Jump RL, Dosa D, LaPlante KL. Antimicrobial stewardship in long-term care facilities: a call to action. J Am Med Dir Assoc. 2016;17(2):183. e1–16.
10. Van Schooneveld T, Miller H, Sayles H, Watkins K, Smith PW. Survey of antimicrobial stewardship practices in Nebraska long-term care facilities. Infect Control Hosp Epidemiol. 2011;32(7):732–4.
11. Morrill HJ, Mermel LA, Baier RR, Alexander-Scott N, Dosa D, Kavoosifar S, et al. Antimicrobial stewardship in Rhode Island long-term care facilities: current standings and future opportunities. Infect Control Hosp Epidemiol. 2016;37(8):979–82.
12. Jump RLP, Gaur S, Katz MJ, Crnich CJ, Dumyati G, Ashraf MS, et al. Template for an antibiotic stewardship policy for post-acute and long-term care settings. J Am Med Dir Assoc. 2017;18(11):913–20.
13. Zarowitz BJ, Allen C, Tangalos E, Ouslander JG. Algorithms promoting antimicrobial stewardship in long-term care. J Am Med Dir Assoc. 2016;17(2):173–8.
14. Jump RL, Olds DM, Seifi N, Kypriotakis G, Jury LA, Peron EP, et al. Effective antimicrobial stewardship in a long-term care facility through an infectious disease consultation service: keeping a LID on antibiotic use. Infect Control Hosp Epidemiol. 2012;33(12):1185–92.
15. Beaulac K, Corcione S, Epstein L, Davidson LE, Doron S. Antimicrobial stewardship in a long-term acute care hospital using offsite electronic medical record audit. Infect Control Hosp Epidemiol. 2016;37(4): 433–9.

16. Kullar R, Yang H, Grein J, Murthy R. A roadmap to implementing anti-microbial stewardship principles in long-term care facilities (LTCFs): collaboration between an acute-care hospital and LTCFs. Clin Infect Dis. 2018;66(8):1304–12.

17. Nicolle LE. Infection prevention issues in long-term care. Curr Opin Infect Dis. 2014;27(4):363–9.

18. Katz MJ, Gurses AP, Tamma PD, Cosgrove SE, Miller MA, Jump RLP. Implementing antimicrobial stewardship in long-term care settings: an integrative review using a human factors approach. Clin Infect Dis. 2017;65(11):1943–51.

19. Brakovich B, Bonham E, VanBrackle L. War on the spore: Clostridium difficile disease among patients in a long-term acute care hospital. J Healthc Qual. 2013;35(3):15–21.

20. Bunch M, Turley J, Johnson K. Antimicrobial stewardship and infection control practices reduced cost and healthcare facility-onset Clostridium difficile infection (HO-CDI) in a long-term acute care (LTAC) setting. Am J Infect Control. 2017;45(6):S18–9.

21. Valiquette L, Cossette B, Garant MP, Diab H, Pepin J. Impact of a reduction in the use of high-risk antibiotics on the course of an epidemic of Clostridium difficile-associated disease caused by the hypervirulent NAP1/027 strain. Clin Infect Dis. 2007;45(Suppl 2):S112–21.

22. Doernberg SB, Dudas V, Trivedi KK. Implementation of an antimicrobial stewardship program targeting residents with urinary tract infections in three community long-term care facilities: a quasi-experimental study using time-series analysis. Antimicrob Resist Infect Control. 2015;4:54.

23. Pate PG, Storey DF, Baum DL. Implementation of an antimicrobial stewardship program at a 60-bed long-term acute care hospital. Infect Control Hosp Epidemiol. 2012;33(4):405–8.

Index

© Springer Nature Switzerland AG 2020   77
T. Chopra (ed.), *Clostridium Difficile Infection in Long-Term Care
Facilities*, https://doi.org/10.1007/978-3-030-29772-5